Asthma

YOUR QUESTIONS ANSWERED

Commissioning Editor: Ellen Green
Project Development Manager: Fiona Conn
Project Manager: Frances Affleck
Design Direction: George Ajayi

Asthma

YOUR QUESTIONS ANSWERED

Antony Crockett
BM MRCGP DRCOG DA
General Practitioner Principal; Clinical Assistant Chest Clinic
Swindon & Marlborough Health Trust, UK

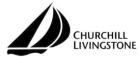

CHURCHILL
LIVINGSTONE

EDINBURGH LONDON NEW YORK PHILADELPHIA ST LOUIS SYDNEY TORONTO 2003

CHURCHILL LIVINGSTONE
An imprint of Elsevier Science Limited

Cover image © imagingbody.com

First published 2003

ISBN 0443 07345 7

British Library Cataloguing in Publication Data
A catalogue record for this book is available from the British Library

Library of Congress Cataloging in Publication Data
A catalog record for this book is available from the Library of Congress

Notice
Medical knowledge is constantly changing. Standard safety precautions must be followed,
but as new research and clinical experience broaden our knowledge, changes in treatment
and drug therapy may become necessary or appropriate. Readers are advised to check the
most current product information provided by the manufacturer of each drug to be
administered to verify the recommended dose, the method and duration of administration,
and contraindications. It is the responsibility of the practitioner, relying on experience and
knowledge of the patient, to determine dosages and the best treatment for each individual
patient. Neither the Publisher nor the author assumes any liability for any injury and/or
damage to persons or property arising from this publication.

 ELSEVIER SCIENCE your source for books,
journals and multimedia
in the health sciences
www.elsevierhealth.com

The
publisher's
policy is to use
paper manufactured
from sustainable forests

Printed in China

Contents

	Preface	vii
	How to use this book	ix
1	What is asthma and who is affected by it?	1
2	Diagnosis of asthma	37
3	Natural history, prognosis and costs of asthma	65
4	Treatment and management of asthma	79
5	Asthma management in practice	161
6	Asthma in the future	223
	Appendix A Drugs and devices used in asthma	231
	Appendix B Devices and drugs currently available in the UK: manufacturers' designs	235
	Appendix C Drugs currently available in the UK that are available as metered-dose inhalers	237
	Appendix D Sources of information	239
	References	247
	Glossary	253
	List of patient questions	255
	Index	257

Preface

Asthma is a very common, chronic disease that affects people of all ages. There is currently no known cure but it can be effectively managed in a variety of ways and most patients should be able to lead a full and active life untroubled by their asthma symptoms or its management.

Over the last twenty or thirty years, our understanding of asthma has greatly increased and our ability to treat it effectively has followed from our understanding. However, it is a very complex, diverse disorder that affects different patients in different ways at different times. We all have lots of unanswered questions about asthma and its management. This book hopes to have posed most of the important questions commonly asked by non-experts (especially general practitioners and practice nurses) about asthma, its management and outcomes; and to have provided up-to-date, relevant and concise answers. It also addresses the problems of organization of asthma care, especially in the community and in general practice, and there is an extensive section providing information about relevant organizations and sources of help, including internet addresses, both in the UK and worldwide. The book is fully referenced and extensively illustrated and the most important clinical points are highlighted.

Nearly all doctors and nurses, and many other healthcare professionals, will have patients who have asthma, sometimes in addition to whatever disorder brings them into contact with their clinician. For that reason we all need to know about asthma and how to manage it successfully. I hope the book provides answers to all the questions a primary care clinician will have, and will help them provide asthma care of the highest standard.

AC

How to use this book

The *Your Questions Answered* series aims to meet the information needs of GPs and other primary care professionals who care for patients with chronic conditions. It is designed to help them work with patients and their families, providing effective, evidence-based care and management.

The books are in an accessible question and answer format, with detailed contents lists at the beginning of every chapter and a complete index to help find specific information.

ICONS

Icons are used in the book to identify particular types of information:

 highlights important information

 highlights side-effect information.

PATIENT QUESTIONS

At the end of relevant chapters there are sections of frequently asked patient questions, with easy-to-understand answers aimed at the non-medical reader. These questions are also listed at the end of the book.

What is asthma and who is affected by it?

1

WHAT IS ASTHMA?

1.1	What is asthma?	4
1.2	What different types of asthma are there?	5
1.3	What is atopic asthma?	5
1.4	What are extrinsic and intrinsic asthma?	5
1.5	What is the difference between a trigger and an allergen?	6
1.6	What are the most common triggers of asthma?	6
1.7	What is the role of viral infections in triggering asthma?	6
1.8	What is the role of the house dust mite in asthma?	7
1.9	What is the role of cats, dogs and other allergens in asthma?	8
1.10	Is oilseed rape a common trigger?	10
1.11	Does exercise trigger asthma?	10
1.12	Does air pollution cause asthma?	11
1.13	Does air pollution make asthma worse?	12
1.14	What is the role of occupational triggers?	13
1.15	What role do non-allergenic triggers play in asthma?	13
1.16	What is the role of passive smoking in asthma?	14
1.17	Is aspirin a common trigger?	14
1.18	Does anxiety or mood affect asthma?	15
1.19	Why is asthma often worse at night?	15
1.20	Can diet worsen asthma?	15
1.21	Can dietary habits cause asthma?	16

CLASSIFICATION AND PREVALENCE OF ASTHMA

1.22	How is asthma classified?	16
1.23	How common is asthma?	17
1.24	How common is asthma in the UK?	17
1.25	Is the prevalence of asthma in the UK high compared with other countries?	19
1.26	Is asthma becoming more common?	19

1.27 Are there any reasons why asthma might be becoming more common? 23

1.28 Could the increase in asthma be due to changes in the indoor environment? 24

1.29 What about the hygiene hypothesis? 25

1.30 Could the increase in asthma be due to changes in the outdoor environment? 25

1.31 Could the increase in asthma be due to changes in diet? 26

1.32 Could the increase in asthma be due to changes in other factors, such as immunity and infections? 26

1.33 Is asthma more common in rural or urban areas? 26

1.34 Are there any stages of life when exposure to allergens is more crucial? 27

1.35 Are there any relevant socioeconomic factors in the development of asthma? 27

WHO GETS ASTHMA?

1.36 Who gets asthma? 27

1.37 Is asthma genetically inherited? 28

1.38 At what age does asthma start? 29

1.39 Is asthma more common in certain races? 29

1.40 Is there a sex bias for asthma? 29

1.41 Can we predict whether a newborn baby will become asthmatic? 29

1.42 Do premature babies have an increased risk of developing asthma? 30

MECHANISM OF ASTHMA

1.43 What is the pathology of asthma? 30

1.44 What is the role of inflammation? 32

1.45 Does it matter at what age sensitization and allergen exposure occur? 33

1.46 What is the effect of the airway inflammation? 33

1.47 Is the inflammation transient or persistent? 34

1.48 What happens in non-allergic asthma? 34

PQ	PATIENT QUESTIONS	
1.49	What is asthma?	35
1.50	Is asthma very common?	35
1.51	Why is asthma becoming more common?	35
1.52	Does pollution cause asthma?	35
1.53	Can you catch asthma?	35
1.54	Can asthma be cured?	36
1.55	If I have asthma, will my baby develop it too?	36

WHAT IS ASTHMA?

1.1 What is asthma?

Asthma is a disease of the airways characterized by inflammation and reversible bronchospasm. It affects people of all ages and races, is very common and has been recognized for thousands of years. Despite huge advances in the knowledge of its pathophysiology, there is no single, universally agreed, definition of asthma. One of the problems of defining asthma is that it is not a single entity but a term used to describe a set of symptoms that result from the action of a number of incompletely understood mechanisms. The common factors are hyperreactive airways that respond to a wide variety of stimuli, reversible airway narrowing, and intermittent, variable symptoms.

The International Consensus Report on diagnosis and management[1] has defined asthma as a chronic inflammatory disorder of the airways in which many cells play a role, including mast cells and eosinophils. In susceptible individuals this inflammation causes symptoms that are usually associated with widespread but variable airflow obstruction that is often reversible either spontaneously or with treatment, and causes an associated increase in airway responsiveness to a variety of stimuli.

The National Institutes of Health Global Initiative for Asthma (GINA) has defined asthma as:[2]

'a chronic inflammatory disorder of the airways. In susceptible individuals this inflammation causes recurrent episodes of wheezing, coughing, chest tightness and difficult breathing. Inflammation makes the airways sensitive to stimuli such as allergens, tobacco smoke, cold air, exercise and chemical irritation. When exposed to stimuli, the airways may become swollen, constricted, filled with mucus and hyperresponsive to a variety of stimuli. The resulting airflow limitation is reversible (although not completely so in some patients), either spontaneously or with treatment. When asthma therapy is adequate inflammation can be reduced over the long term, symptoms can be controlled and most asthma-related problems prevented' (p. 1).

This definition emphasizes the importance of inflammation in the aetiology of asthma, and also the fact that the inflammation causes the airways to be hypersensitive to external stimuli, and not vice versa. This definition also correctly suggests that proper management is possible and desirable.

A more pragmatic definition applicable in primary care is that asthma is characterized by the periodic occurrence of one or more of the following symptoms established by taking a patient's medical history: wheezing, dyspnoea or coughing, combined with one or more of the following objective criteria: reversible airway obstruction or clinical peak flow variability of more than 20%.

However, this is still difficult to remember. The definition below is, above all, very simple:

> Asthma is a disease of the respiratory system involving inflammation of the airways and reversible symptoms and signs of bronchospasm.

1.2   What different types of asthma are there?

■ Allergic asthma is characterized by an allergic response involving airway inflammation resulting from exposure of the susceptible individual to certain specific triggers such as animal dander, pollen or dust.

■ Atopic asthma is a specific type of allergic asthma involving an immunoglobulin (Ig) E-mediated reaction. It is most common in children; other manifestations of atopy include allergic dermatitis and allergic rhinitis (hay fever). Although this classification is appropriate from a pathological viewpoint, it is less useful for clinicians.

1.3   What is atopic asthma?

Atopic asthma describes a particular type of allergic asthma involving an exaggerated immune response that includes IgE activation and mast cell degradation. Other manifestations of atopy include allergic rhinitis, allergic conjunctivitis and atopic dermatitis. Nearly all allergic asthma is atopic.

1.4   What are extrinsic and intrinsic asthma?

EXTRINSIC ASTHMA

Extrinsic asthma is asthma triggered by an external allergen, such as pollen, animals or house dust mites; exposure to such triggers sets off an allergic reaction culminating in the symptoms and signs of asthma. The allergic reaction usually involves IgE and is therefore atopic. Childhood asthma is usually extrinsic. People with extrinsic asthma may have asthma of varying severity and symptoms that are provoked by a variety of triggers, not all of which are allergens.

INTRINSIC ASTHMA

Intrinsic asthma is asthma that occurs in a person who is not atopic, and is more common in asthma that starts in adults. Triggers are usually non-specific, such as viral infections, changes in temperature or humidity, and smoke or dust. Allergies to external allergens such as pollen and house dust mites are not a feature of intrinsic asthma. There is no difference between extrinsic and intrinsic asthma in the histology of the airways or in response to treatment with corticosteroids.

TRIGGERS AND ALLERGENS

1.5 What is the difference between a trigger and an allergen?

All allergens are triggers but not all triggers are allergens:

■ A *trigger* is any substance that is capable of inducing or exacerbating asthma. Examples include cold air, exercise and viral upper respiratory tract infections.
■ An *allergen* is a special form or type of trigger that induces allergic asthma. Examples include cat dander, pollen and house dust mites.
■ An *allergic reaction* or *allergy* describes a type of immune response to external agents in which the response itself causes harm or damage to the body.

There is a strong association between allergy and asthma. In order to establish that a specific allergen causes an effect, it is necessary to demonstrate that exposure to that allergen leads to an increase in asthmatic symptoms.

1.6 What are the most common triggers of asthma?

COMMON ASTHMA TRIGGERS

Common triggers, in descending order of importance (this is an objective list, for which there is evidence), are:

■ Infections
■ *Allergens* – house dust mites, animal dander, fungi, pollens
■ Exercise
■ Environmental pollutants
■ Cold air
■ Occupational agents
■ Hyperventilation.

1.7 What is the role of viral infections in triggering asthma?

Acute upper respiratory tract viral infections are among the commonest triggers of both intrinsic and (especially) extrinsic asthma. Most are rhinoviruses, which give symptoms of the common cold and cause acute inflammatory rhinitis. The rhinitis results in the release of mediators from the nasal mucosa; these mediators worsen the rhinitis and also have the potential to cause bronchospasm in asthmatic individuals. The viral infection also results in eosinophil recruitment within the lower airways. These eosinophils will release mediators, which in turn lead to bronchoconstriction and increased mucus secretion. Viral infection of nasal epithelial cells therefore results in worsening of the eosinophilic airway inflammation in asthma and deterioration in asthma control.

Asthma is more common in children who have had croup or other lower respiratory infections in early life. There is an association between early respiratory illness (before the age of 2 years, severe enough to require treatment by a doctor) and the later development of asthma. It may be that the undiagnosed asthma was the cause of the respiratory infection in early life rather than the effect of it. Viral infections in the absence of atopy do not appear to be risk factors for the development of asthma. Infection with the bacterium *Chlamydia pneumoniae* has been implicated in new-onset asthma and in the pathogenesis of chronic stable asthma. However, treatment with appropriate antibiotics provides no significant long-term benefit.

1.8 What is the role of the house dust mite in asthma?

One of the most common allergens in the UK – and indeed worldwide – is the house dust mite (*Fig. 1.1*). These tiny creatures eat human skin scales that have been shed. They live, breed and die in our homes. It is not the mite itself that is the allergen, but particles it excretes that contain the

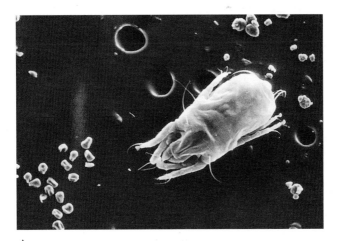

▲
Fig. 1.1 The house dust mite is ubiquitous and difficult to eradicate. It is a potent trigger of asthma for many people, especially those with atopy. From Roitt I, Brostoff J, Male D (eds.) (2001) *Immunology*, 6th edn. Edinburgh: Mosby, with permission.

allergens Der p1, Der p2 and Der p3. It is now known that variations in house dust mite concentration correlate closely with changes in bronchial responses. House dust mites like foam-backed carpets, a square metre of which may harbour up to 1.5 million mites. House dust mites and their waste make up one-third of all dust from carpets, and a feather pillow may contain 60 million mites weighing 90 grams. The concentration of mite allergen in most homes in the UK has increased fourfold in the past 10 years. There are, therefore, huge quantities of house dust mite allergen in our home environments.

Exposure of susceptible individuals to house dust mites causes bronchospasm within 15 minutes, with inflammation and oedema of the airways. The critical period of a child's life when sensitization to the house dust mite allergen occurs is the first year, when the mucosal immune system is still overreactive, or in the second and third trimester of intrauterine life. The higher the level of allergen, the greater the likelihood of the child developing asthma.

Other non-allergic factors such as tobacco smoke, air pollution or viral infection may influence this sensitization process. House dust mite concentration in schools, however, appears to be lower than in homes. Carpeted floors increase exposure to house dust mites at school but, even so, house dust mite is unlikely to cause problems for allergic children at school as the levels are rarely high enough.

The vast majority of children with allergic asthma will have a positive result on skin prick testing for house dust mite allergen.

1.9 What is the role of cats, dogs and other allergens in asthma?

■ Cats and dogs are also important allergic triggers of asthma. The critical concentration is about 8 micrograms of cat or dog allergen per gram of dust.

■ Cats are common pets in the UK (*Fig. 1.2*). About 3% of the population is allergic to cats and up to 40% of children with asthma are sensitized to cat allergens, making it the second most important allergen after house dust mite in childhood asthma.

■ The cat allergen is thought to be in the skin of the cat, not in the saliva as was once believed. Traces of clinically relevant allergen can be found up to 3 months after a cat has vacated a room. Cats should be completely banned from the bedrooms of any child whose asthma is severe or is made worse by exposure to cats.

■ Dog allergen may be a major cause of asthma but has received less attention than cat allergen in recent years. However, dog ownership is often linked to poorer domestic hygiene and to larger families, and these two factors are associated with lower rates of asthma.

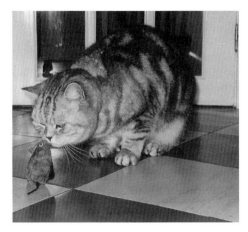

◀ **Fig. 1.2** Traces of cat dander are found even in households that have never owned one. It takes many months for all traces of cat allergens to disappear, even if the cat is no longer present.

■ Both cat and dog allergens can be found in samples of dust collected from public transport and public buildings. Sometimes the concentrations in these places are higher than in cat- or dog-owning households. Curtains, mattresses, sofas and soft toys are also important reservoirs for dog and cat allergens.

■ Other important allergens include fungi and moulds, pollens and cockroaches. Many asthmatics, especially those who are atopic, will be sensitive to the spring and summer pollens (*Fig. 1.3*), but a significant number are sensitive to moulds and fungal spores, which are more prevalent in the autumn and winter months.

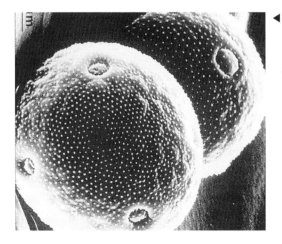

◀ **Fig. 1.3** Many pollen particles are too large to cause bronchial allergy (they are filtered by the nose), but there are many asthmatics whose symptoms are readily triggered by a variety of common pollens, such as grasses.

1.10   Is oilseed rape a common trigger?

Some patients unfairly blame other perceived triggers. Oilseed rape is easy to see and smell in the early summer (*Fig. 1.4*), and is blamed by many asthmatics for any worsening of their symptoms. However, a close study of people who blamed oilseed rape found that subjects were in fact rarely allergic to it and fewer than half were atopic.[3] Such patients may well be allergic to other allergens, including other grasses and plants that release their pollen at the same time, especially Timothy grass (a potent allergen and often found growing in the verges of fields containing oilseed rape), or their asthma may be worsened by chemicals released by the crop or rising summer ozone levels. What is clear, however, is that oilseed rape is innocent.

1.11   Does exercise trigger asthma?

The majority of asthmatics have worsening symptoms on or after physical activity. Exercise of reasonable intensity causes a small amount of bronchodilatation in normal subjects and in some asthmatics, but intense exercise for at least 6 minutes results in bronchoconstriction in most

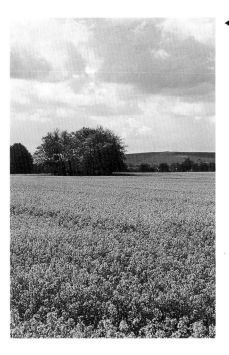

◀ **Fig. 1.4** Oilseed rape. This crop is increasingly farmed in Europe and North America. It has a bright yellow colour and striking aroma, but is unfairly blamed for triggering asthma – its particle size is far too big to enter the lungs.

asthmatics. The bronchospasm and accompanying symptoms occur 5–15 minutes after the end of the exercise and may last for 30–40 minutes, although it may recur in a minority of asthmatics some hours later. The characteristic of exercise-induced asthma that distinguishes it from other causes of exercise-induced breathlessness is that the breathlessness continues for some time after the exercise has finished only in exercise-induced asthma. Running and cycling appear to be more provocative than swimming. The trigger is thought to be the cooling and drying of the airways subsequent to hyperventilation that occurs on exertion. The drying of the airway mucosa leads to mediator release and bronchospasm. For a few asthmatics, exercise-induced symptoms may be the only manifestation of their asthma.

1.12   Does air pollution cause asthma?

Most of the public and the non-medical press seem to be fairly convinced that pollution is a major cause of asthma and is one of the main reasons that asthma is becoming more common and more severe. However, there is no clear evidence linking air pollution with increasing asthma prevalence or severity. While the association of outdoor air pollution with increased prevalence and severity of other respiratory diseases and heart diseases is well known, for asthma there are few supporting data. This is true whether one considers particulate pollution, which derives mostly from vehicle exhausts, or pollution arising from the burning of fossil fuels. Non-particulate pollution describes chemicals such as sulfur dioxide, ozone and nitrous oxide. These chemicals certainly enhance the response of the asthmatic to inhaled allergens, but by themselves do not cause asthma.

Again, despite popular prejudice, there is no increase in the risk of developing asthma from living close to a busy road (*Fig. 1.5*). A study comparing the frequency and severity of asthma in urban Newcastle with that in rural Cumbria[4] found no evidence to implicate the role of pollution in the perceived recent increase in asthma prevalence. The unification of Germany allowed two populations of similar genetic stock, geography and climate to be compared.[5] People living in the former West Germany were exposed to relatively low levels of outdoor atmospheric pollution whereas those of the former East had relatively high levels, especially of particulates and sulfur dioxide. For the children studied, the prevalence of asthma and hay fever was much higher in the relatively unpolluted former West Germany, whereas the prevalence of bronchitis and bronchiolitis was much higher in the polluted former East Germany. Atmospheric air pollution is therefore associated with respiratory disease, but not definitely with asthma. Indeed, while asthma prevalence in the UK has increased over the past 20 years, levels of sulfur dioxide and black smoke have actually decreased as a result of the Clean Air Acts. The prevalence of asthma is no greater in urban

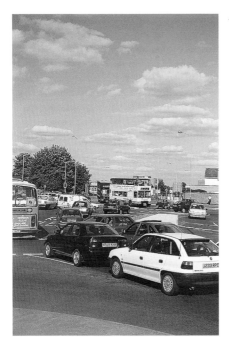

◄ **Fig. 1.5** Exposure to road traffic fumes is popularly assumed to be a major factor in any increase in the severity or prevalence of asthma, but there is little scientific evidence to support this.

areas than in rural areas, nor in people exposed occupationally to traffic such as traffic police. This evidence is further borne out by European studies that do not show higher incidences of atopy and asthmatic symptoms in Polish children exposed to pollution at higher levels than their Swedish counterparts. The highest prevalence of asthma in the UK in children is on the Isle of Skye,[6] which surely must be one of the least polluted parts of the country. Similarly Australia and New Zealand have very high prevalence rates of asthma but are among the least polluted parts of the world.

1.13 Does air pollution make asthma worse?

Asthmatics are more likely to be sensitive to air pollutants such as sulfur dioxide, ozone and nitrogen oxides; pollutants may also enhance the response to allergens, and the net affect of inhaled atmospheric pollutants may therefore be greater because a subject has worse lung function initially. Some patients may be made worse by some types of pollution, but the effect is small for the general population. Even living in an area exposed to volcanic ash particles made little difference to asthma symptoms or medication use in a large study in New Zealand.[7] Patients with severe asthma may, however, find that their disease worsens on days when pollution is high, but the effect of high levels of pollution will be more marked for those who are suffering from non-asthmatic, chronic respiratory diseases (especially chronic obstructive pulmonary disease) and heart disease than for patients with asthma.

In summary, pollution has a small or no part to play in making asthma more common or more severe. However, the idea of pollution causing asthma and making asthma worse has certainly taken root in the public psyche, and the idea is supported by the vast majority of the non-medical press.

1.14   What is the role of occupational triggers?

Occupational asthma occurs when exposure to agents at work results in an individual becoming asthmatic. Subsequent exposure will provoke further episodes of asthma. About 5% of all adult cases of asthma are thought to be related (at least in part) to occupation. Atopic individuals are more likely to develop occupational asthma, more so to agents of high molecular weight (such as animal products) than to those of lower molecular weight (such as isocyanates). If the diagnosis is made late or the patient has severe disease, asthma symptoms may persist even after removal from the offending environmental agent. Occupational agents can induce airway inflammation, bronchial hyperreactivity and symptoms of asthma. This airway response differs from and must be distinguished from inciters of asthma that may be commonly encountered in the workplace, such as exercise, general dust or damp, by people with previously diagnosed asthma.

Occupational asthma is discussed more fully in Q. 5.61–5.66. *Table 1.1* shows the agents that can commonly cause occupational asthma.

1.15   What role do non-allergenic triggers play in asthma?

By far and away the commonest triggers of acute asthma exacerbations, especially in school-aged children, are upper respiratory tract infections. Other important triggers appear to be living in damp houses and thunderstorms. Children of families that use wood or coal for heating and cooking have a significantly lower prevalence of hay fever, atopy and asthma than children living in homes with other heating systems. Whether this is due to factors directly related to wood or coal combustion, or to the use of such fuels as a marker of different lifestyles, is not clear.

The latest survey in the UK[8] listed the following factors as being important in affecting the respondents' asthma, the most common being quoted first (this is a subjective list of perceived important triggers):

■ Viruses or colds
■ Changes in the weather

TABLE 1.1 Common causative agents of occupational asthma

Causative agent	Main occupations
Isocyanates	Plastics industry, paint industry (especially polyurethanes), those who work with varnishes, adhesives or printing
Grain and flour	Bakers, farmers, millers
Animals, including insects and larvae	Laboratory workers, pest controllers, fruit cultivators
Epoxy resins	Workers in the plastics, adhesives and paints industries; workers in paint manufacturing
Wood dusts	Carpenters, timber industry
Cholophany	Workers in the electronics industry, especially where rosin is used as a soldering flux
Glutaraldehyde	Nurses, laboratory staff, radiographers, radiologists
Proteolytic enzymes	Workers who manufacture washing powders; workers in the baking, brewing and leather industries
Drugs (e.g. antibiotics, cimetidine, ipecacuanha, ispaghula dust)	Pharmaceutical workers, nurses
Dyes	Workers in textile manufacturing industries
Soya, tea, coffee dust	Food processors
Castor bean dust	Merchant seamen, laboratory workers, felt makers

- ■ Areas with heavy pollution
- ■ Smoky atmosphere
- ■ Exercise or activity
- ■ Pollen
- ■ Stress
- ■ Pets.

1.16 What is the role of passive smoking in asthma?

There is increasing evidence that passive smoking is involved in the aetiology of childhood asthma – to a small extent. Children born to mothers who smoked in pregnancy will have raised cord blood IgE levels (*see Q. 1.41*) as well as a reduced birthweight and airway size. Many studies have shown that parental smoking is a small but consistent risk factor for children having recurrent respiratory infections, which in themselves may be an important factor in later developing asthma. The risks from passive smoking appear to be greater in lower socioeconomic groups.

1.17 Is aspirin a common trigger?

About 10% of asthmatics will be sensitive to aspirin: their asthma is made suddenly worse after taking aspirin. Patients known to be sensitive should studiously avoid all aspirin, aspirin products and aspirin-related products such as the non-steroidal anti-inflammatory drugs (NSAIDs) (e.g. ibuprofen). They should be cautious when buying over-the-counter medicines, and if they are in any doubt they should consult their doctor or pharmacist. Aspirin-sensitive asthma is rarely seen in children, even where there is no general ban on prescribing aspirin to children aged under 12 years. Asthmatics who are known not to be aspirin sensitive can safely use aspirin and aspirin-related products.

Asthmatics who are unsure whether their asthma can be triggered by aspirin should avoid NSAIDs and aspirin if they also have other manifestations of allergic disorders. Examples include nasal polyps, allergic rhinitis or conjunctivitis, rhinorrhoea, anosmia, dietary sensitivity or persistent asthma needing frequent or continuous oral steroids. *See also Q. 5.92.*

1.18 Does anxiety or mood affect asthma?

Asthma may often be made worse with changes in mood or psychological or psychiatric states, but these are not true triggers. A number of asthmatics will respond to small changes in airway resistance by hyperventilating, leading to worsening dyspnoea and increased symptoms, despite little objective evidence of worsening asthma. Similar responses occur in some asthmatics when they laugh or cry.

There is an increased risk of death from asthma in patients with severe depression, recent bereavement or unemployment, alcohol abuse and schizophrenia. Asthma can – and often does – lead to low self-esteem and low self-confidence, and to panic attacks. *See Q. 3.8.*

1.19 Why is asthma often worse at night?

Many asthmatics experience worse symptoms at night, especially during times when their asthma is worse anyway, but night is not a true trigger.

Many patients with poorly controlled asthma may have nocturnal symptoms. The cause is not fully established, but may involve the effects of increased vagal tone. Airway inflammation is also increased at night and this will contribute to airway narrowing. Again, the cause of increased airway inflammation at night is not known.

1.20 Can diet worsen asthma?

For the majority of asthmatics, dietary factors are neither the cause of their asthma nor significant triggers for worsening asthma. Certain foods may trigger asthma exacerbations in a few susceptible patients, but individual foods or food products are often quite difficult to identify and asthma triggered only by food is extremely rare.

Some atopic asthmatics may have an IgE-dependent reaction in response to ingesting specific foods, resulting in a type I hypersensitivity reaction. Such foods include shellfish, nuts and fruits such as bananas, kiwi and avocado, which all contain molecules related to latex. The hypersensitivity reaction may produce urticaria, rhinitis and anaphylaxis as well as an asthmatic response. Cross-reactions between allergens in foods and allergens present in the air can also occur, and the reaction is also an IgE-mediated type I hypersensitivity. A good example is the birch pollen allergy syndrome. Birch pollen is a common cause of hay fever but it can also be found in some apples and pears. When eaten raw, these fruits may contain sufficient cross-reacting allergen to induce an acute asthma episode.

Other asthmatics may experience problems after eating certain foods where the mechanism is not mediated via IgE but by histamine. Histamine is an important mediator of allergic reactions and high concentrations can be released by mature cheeses or certain fish species, especially if not fresh, causing an acute asthma episode in susceptible individuals. Other foods (e.g. strawberries) cause the release of histamine from mast cells via a non-IgE-mediated reaction.

There is another group of chemicals that can cause non-IgE-mediated acute reactions to food as a result of a variety of ill-understood mechanisms. These include drugs such as aspirin (*see also* Q. 5.92) as well as food additives such as sodium metabisulfite (found in red wine especially) and tartrazine.

1.21 Can dietary habits cause asthma?

Diet may be responsible for some of the differences in the prevalence rates of asthma between countries, but the details of which dietary factors are significant are not known.

One hypothesis is that a fall in the dietary intake of antioxidants (mainly vitamins A, C and E, found in fresh fruit and vegetables) leads to increased airway sensitivity in response to injury. This view is consistent with the hypothesis that the observed reduction in antioxidant intake in the British diet over the past 25 years has been a factor in the increased prevalence of asthma in this period. The increased risk of developing symptoms has also been linked to low levels of zinc, vitamin C, manganese and magnesium in the diet.

CLASSIFICATION AND PREVALENCE OF ASTHMA

1.22 How is asthma classified?

In practice, it is more usual to classify asthma by its severity, irrespective of the aetiology. The severity of asthma is, in turn, often measured by the amounts and types of medication needed to control the symptoms.

The British Thoracic Society (BTS)–Scottish Intercollegiate Guidelines Network (SIGN)[9] guidelines use five grades or steps:

- *Step 1* includes 'trivial' and potential. This category is asthma that can be controlled adequately by intermittent treatment, taken as needed.
- *Step 2* describes asthma that is adequately controlled by regular inhaled anti-inflammatory treatment (usually inhaled steroids).
- *Step 3* describes asthma that is adequately controlled by regular inhaled anti-inflammatory treatment plus regular inhaled long-acting β_2-agonists.
- *Step 4* describes asthma that requires step 3 treatment together with additional therapies.
- *Step 5* describes asthma that requires chronic oral steroid treatment.

In the UK, most clinicians use the BTS classification. The GINA classification is more widely used elsewhere, especially in the USA and Canada. GINA classifies asthma into four grades of severity:

- Mild, including 'trivial' and potential
- Moderate intermittent
- Moderate persistent
- Severe.

1.23 How common is asthma?

Asthma is a common disease throughout the world. GINA[10] estimates that there are over 150 million people worldwide who have asthma. In the USA there are 9–12 million sufferers. Prevalence rates vary markedly between different countries, in part accounted for by differing diagnostic approaches. The prevalence of recent wheeze in 7–11-year-olds varies from 25% in Chile to 1% in China.

The International Study of Asthma and Allergies in Childhood (ISAAC) reported in 1998,[11] and found that asthma was becoming more common, especially in northern and western Europe, Australasia and North America (*Table 1.2*). Low prevalence rates were found in southern Europe, most tropical countries and Iceland and Norway. Intermediate rates were found in Eastern Europe. Countries where low levels of symptoms were reported included Indonesia, Greece, China, Taiwan, Uzbekistan, India and Ethiopia.

1.24 How common is asthma in the UK?

A figure commonly given for the prevalence of asthma in the UK is 5% of adults and 10% of children. However, more recent surveys, such as the 2001 National Asthma Campaign Audit performed in the UK,[8] indicate that over

TABLE 1.2 International comparisons of the prevalence of asthma and wheeze in children aged 13–14 years

Country	Wheeze last year (%)	≥ 4 wheeze attacks last year (%)	Ever diagnosed asthma (%)
Highest prevalence			
Australia	29.4	10.0	28.2
Peru	26.0	4.8	28.0
New Zealand	30.2	9.9	24.4
Singapore	9.7	2.1	20.9
UK	32.2	9.3	20.7
Lowest prevalence			
South Korea	7.7	1.6	2.4
Russia	4.4	0.7	2.4
Uzbekistan	9.2	0.7	1.7
Indonesia	2.1	0.4	1.6
Albania	2.6	0.3	1.6

From National Asthma Campaign 2001[7], with permission.

15% of children and 7% of adults will have been given a diagnosis of asthma in their lifetime – some 8 million people.

The prevalence of diagnosed asthma is higher in children than in adults (*Fig. 1.6*). By combining the findings of asthma prevalence studies in specific

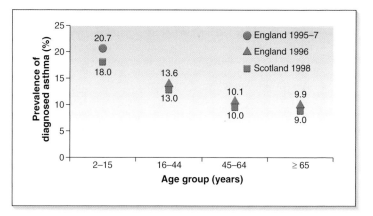

Fig. 1.6 Age-specific prevalence of diagnosed asthma in England and Scotland. The prevalence of asthma is higher in children than in adults. From National Asthma Campaign 2001,[8] with permission.

age groups and applying the subsequent results to the latest UK demographic data, there are about 5.1 million people in the UK currently receiving treatment for asthma: 3.7 million adults and 1.4 million children.

Prevalence rates also vary in different locations in the UK, with particularly high rates in the islands and highlands of Scotland and in the Oxford and Anglia regions of England. However, the prevalence of diagnosed asthma is slightly lower for children in Scotland than in England, but similar for all other age groups.

1.25   Is the prevalence of asthma in the UK high compared with other countries?

The ISAAC study found that countries with the highest prevalence of asthma symptoms reported in the preceding 12 months were Australia, New Zealand, UK and Ireland, followed by centres in the USA, Canada and Latin America. The UK has the highest rate in Europe for young adults aged 20–44 years reporting current symptoms and use of medication for asthma.

1.26   Is asthma becoming more common?

Incidence

The incidence of asthma is difficult to quantify, as current measures of asthma cannot separate first diagnoses of asthma from new episodes of asthma in patients already diagnosed. What is known is that the number of new or first asthma episodes presenting to general practitioners (GPs) has increased considerably in the past 20–30 years, peaking in about 1993, and slowly declining since (*Fig. 1.7*). The increase is especially marked in pre-school children, again peaking in 1993 when the number of new or first asthma episodes in this age group was 11 times greater than the number of episodes reported in the mid-1970s. The weekly incidence of asthma episodes is currently 3–4 times higher in adults and 6 times higher in children compared with 25 years ago. Recent data published by the National Asthma Campaign's 2001 Audit[8] show that new episodes of asthma occur most commonly in young children, as a proportion of their age group, and the relative proportions decline slightly in older age groups (*Fig. 1.8*).

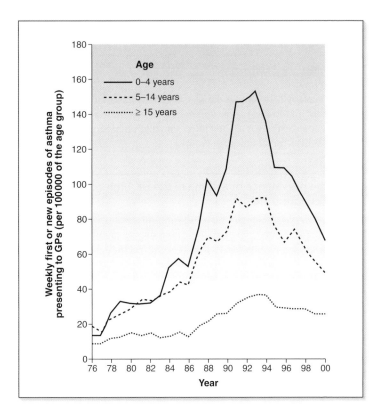

▲

Fig. 1.7 Average weekly first episodes of asthma presenting to general practitioners (GPs) in England and Wales, 1976–2000. The incidence of asthma episodes presented to GPs has increased considerably over the past 25 years, particularly in children, but now seems to be decreasing again. From National Asthma Campaign 2001,[8] with permission.

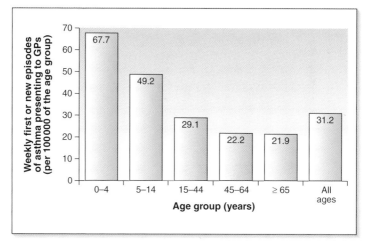

▲

Fig. 1.8 Average weekly incidence of asthma episodes presenting to general practitioners (GPs) in England and Wales in 2000. The incidence of asthma is particularly high among children. From National Asthma Campaign 2001,[8] with permission.

Prevalence

Asthma is very common at all ages and is becoming more common in children and adults, especially in the last 20–30 years. The prevalence of wheeze in adults increased by 5% between 1991 and 1996 (*Fig. 1.9*). The prevalence of wheeze in children also increased between 1990 and 1998, as did the prevalence of children with diagnosed asthma (*Fig. 1.10*). The reason for this increase is uncertain, but is probably due to a variety of interacting factors, such as exposure to smoking, indoor and outdoor pollution, genetic susceptibility and diet, rather than to one single cause. The timing of exposure to certain triggers at certain ages in certain individuals is also important. Some of the increase in reported wheeze can be accounted for by patient or doctor factors. Many patients will report a history of symptoms that may not be due to asthma at all, and indeed their recollection of their own or their children's symptoms may be inaccurate. There may also be a greater willingness for patients to report symptoms and for doctors to act on them than previously.

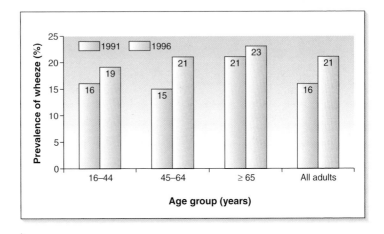

Fig. 1.9 Age-specific trends in the prevalence of wheeze in adults in England, 1991–1996. The prevalence in England increased by 5% between 1991 and 1996. From National Asthma Campaign 2001,[8] with permission.

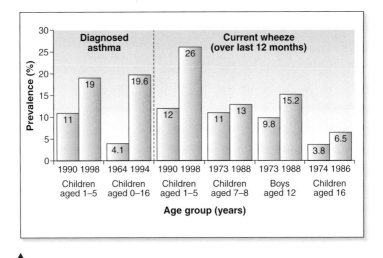

Fig. 1.10 Trends in the prevalence of asthma and wheeze from repeat prevalence studies in the UK. The prevalence in children has increased during the past three decades. From National Asthma Campaign 2001,[8] with permission.

Overall, the consensus is that the prevalence of asthma is rising and that the increase is real. Evidence to support a real rise in asthma prevalence comes indirectly from the observations that there are increasing rates of other atopic conditions (e.g. atopic dermatitis and hay fever) measured over the same period for which the rates of wheezing and asthma have been reported as rising. Of course, it may be that doctors and patients are once again taking more notice of conditions whose prevalence is actually static.

Statistics from general practice in the UK show that the age-standardized prevalence of treated asthma per 1000 patients increased from 67.5 to 73.2 in males and from 67.1 to 76.5 in females between 1994 and 1998.

1.27   Are there any reasons why asthma might be becoming more common?

POSSIBLE EXPLANATIONS FOR THE INCREASE IN ASTHMA PREVALENCE

The prevalence of asthma in children has been increasing for some time, and is still increasing, especially in Europe, North America and Australasia. A worldwide review of 16 repeated surveys of the rising prevalence of asthma in children and young adults concluded that increased professional and public awareness of asthma might be responsible for some of the increase in diagnosis. Only one study reported any increase in an objective measurement. Repeated surveys incorporating more objective data are needed before firm conclusions about any continuing increase in asthma can be drawn. In adults, on the other hand, the prevalence of asthma is more stable, or, when it is found to be increasing, the increase is among those with the mildest symptoms.

There has been an increase not only in the prevalence of childhood asthma, but also in the prevalence of other atopic disorders. Why this should be is unclear and there is no single cause. Theories for the increasing prevalence of asthma include:

- *The indoor pollutant hypothesis*: better-insulated homes with central heating and fitted carpets have led to an increase in house dust mite and cockroach populations.
- *The hygiene hypothesis*: children raised on farms, or in households where hygiene may not be meticulous, or with dogs, tend to have lower rates of asthma. Having many siblings also seems to reduce the rates of asthma.
- *The outdoor pollutant hypothesis*: increased exposure to particulate pollutants, especially diesel fumes, chemicals or ozone has led to an increase in asthma.
- *The dietary hypothesis*: over the past 10–30 years, there has been a tendency to eat and drink more processed foods (and chemical additives) and less fresh fruit and vegetables (containing antioxidants),

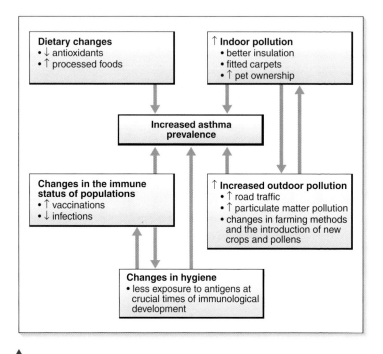

▲

Fig. 1.11 Factors associated with the increasing prevalence of asthma over the past decade.

polyunsaturated fats and fish. Asthma rates have increased more in societies where this dietary trend is strongest.

■ *The immune hypothesis*: over the past two or three decades rates of infectious diseases, especially in childhood, have fallen dramatically in the developed world, partly due to widespread use of vaccines. Changes in the immune status of whole populations may account for the increase in asthma and perhaps other disorders such as rheumatoid arthritis and diabetes.

A combination of factors is more than likely than a single one. *Fig. 1.11* summarizes these theories.

1.28 **Could the increase in asthma be due to changes in the indoor environment?**

In most Western countries, the majority of people lead more sedentary lives than in previous generations, and spend more time indoors. Their homes are warmer and usually have central heating, and gas rather than solid fuel fires. Home insulation has improved, so air changes may be as low as 0.2 changes per hour (laboratory rats are required to have 10 changes per hour). As a result of these changes, there are greater amounts of immunologically foreign proteins derived from indoor sources (such as house dust mites and cockroaches) in the indoor air. Inhalation of such allergens can sensitize and affect the immune response of genetically predisposed individuals.

The increase in allergic disorders may also be due to an increase in the total allergen load, especially from house dust mites and cats.

Indoor environmental allergens are very important, especially house dust mites and cats, but these factors alone probably do not account for the known increases in diagnosed asthma.

1.29 What about the hygiene hypothesis?

Over the past 20–30 years, people have been living much more hygienically and inhabiting cleaner houses and public buildings. In addition, the immune response itself may have changed in the last few generations owing to the more widespread use of antibiotics, or to immunization against previously common infectious diseases such as whooping cough. One hypothesis is that populations who were previously exposed to high levels of infections such as tuberculosis were protected from reacting to allergens, whereas now their lymphocytes are relatively idle and free to act against allergens at an early age, leading to atopy. Some evidence for this hypothesis comes from Germany, where higher levels of asthma were reported in children living in towns than on farms.

1.30 Could the increase in asthma be due to changes in the outdoor environment?

There are three main outdoor environmental factors important in asthma: the weather, outdoor pollution, and aeroallergens such as pollen and spores. All three may overlap and affect the influence of the others.

Many asthmatics notice that their asthma control is sensitive to changes in the weather. Asthma is often more troublesome when temperatures drop in the autumn, or when there are thunderstorms.

Pollens are a potent cause of hay fever but are also important in allergic asthma. The particles of many pollens are too large to be inhaled into the bronchi (see Q. 1.10). Spores tend to be much smaller and are therefore more likely to be implicated in many people's allergic asthma, especially if their asthma tends to be more severe in the autumn.

Outdoor pollution can be a trigger for asthma but is unlikely to be the only cause. Indeed, the recent rise in the frequency of asthma coincides with a fall in the atmospheric concentration of fossil fuel combustion products, mainly sulfur dioxide and particulates. However, exposure to pollutants in infancy may affect bronchial hyperreactivity. A Norwegian study compared children who had lived all their lives in one of two valleys, one of which was polluted by an aluminium smelter. The risk of developing bronchial hyperreactivity at school-age increased with exposure to the pollutants in the first three years of life. The role of pollution is discussed more fully in *Q. 1.12 and Q. 1.13*

1.31 Could the increase in asthma be due to changes in diet?

Another hypothesis is that a fall in dietary intakes of antioxidants (mainly vitamins A, C and E, found in fresh fruit and vegetables) leads to increased airway sensitivity to injury. This view is consistent with the hypothesis that the observed reduction in antioxidant intake in the British diet over the past 25 years has been a factor in the increase in the prevalence of asthma in this period. The increased risk of developing symptoms has also been linked to low levels of zinc, vitamin C, manganese and magnesium in the diet. *See Q. 1. 20 and Q. 1.21*

1.32 Could the increase in asthma be due to changes in other factors, such as immunity and infections?

Since the 1960s most children in the developed world have received many immunizations against such diseases as polio and whooping cough. In addition, many children will have had several courses of antibiotic therapy, usually for ear, throat and chest symptoms. Could these events affect the risks of developing asthma? This theory is supported by research that has highlighted the role of helper T lymphocyte cells in the immunopathogenesis of asthma. Repeated exposure of the body to external organisms will cause the T helper cells to differentiate into type 1 cells (Th1), which form part of the normal immune response to viruses, bacteria and fungi. The production of Th1 cells also inhibits the T helper cells from differentiating into type 2 cells (Th2), which have a key role in the mechanism of airway inflammation. Lack of exposure to external pathogens results in relative excess Th2 production and to asthma.[12]

1.33 Is asthma more common in rural or urban areas?

Asthma is slightly more common in urban than in rural areas. The highest prevalence occurred in suburban areas, rather than the inner city. Factors such as industrial pollution or road traffic density appear to be less important than environmental triggers such as pollens and moulds. Microclimate conditions prevailing in the atmosphere over outer urban areas will attract and hold higher levels of pollen and organic material than can be found in the atmospheres over rural or inner-city areas. The areas with the highest incidences of asthma in the UK are the Scottish islands and highlands, and in the world are in New Zealand and Australia.[11]

1.34 Are there any stages of life when exposure to allergens is more crucial?

There may also be changes in the airway responsiveness of populations as a whole. These airway responses are triggered by the exposure of susceptible individuals to specific allergens or combinations of allergens at a critical time in their immunological development. The critical times for sensitization to new allergens appear to be early infancy and young adulthood. Maternal smoking and maternal exposure to allergens (especially house dust mite and cats) during pregnancy increases the resulting child's later immune responsiveness.

1.35 Are there any relevant socioeconomic factors in the development of asthma?

■ Asthma is more common in poorer people at all age groups.
■ Asthma also tends to be more severe in poorer people.
■ The mortality rates for asthma tend to be higher in poorer people.

Explanations include:

■ Dietary influences: less fresh fruit and vegetables and oily fish consumption, and higher saturated fats.
■ Housing influences: relative overcrowding.
■ Poorer people tend to access health care less appropriately and less promptly.

WHO GETS ASTHMA?

1.36 Who gets asthma?

There is undoubtedly a genetic component to asthma, but it is by no means an inherited disorder. A child born to two atopic parents has about a 66% chance of developing one or more atopic phenotypes; a child with one atopic parent has a 33% risk of such a development. There is a strong environmental component in addition, as evidenced by the fact that immigrants from countries with low rates of asthma, such as much of Africa, to countries with higher rates, such as western Europe or Australasia, will show an increased rate of asthma with time. Similar evidence also comes from rising rates of asthma in cities or countries where affluence is increasing among people of stable genetic stock.

1.37   Is asthma genetically inherited?

■ It is obvious to anybody working with asthmatics that asthma tends to run in families, and especially so in families with a strong history of allergies and atopy. It is likely that some individuals are genetically predisposed to having hypersensitive airways and therefore to developing allergic asthma. It appears that there may be different genetic linkages for the atopic IgE-mediated response and a different gene that influences bronchial hyperreactivity even in the absence of atopy.

■ There are many genes associated with the development of asthma and atopy, and these genes are widely distributed throughout the world, in all races and communities. There are far more people with one or more genes associated with atopy than there are people who have clinical allergies.

■ Studies of twins have suggested that a genetic factor confers susceptibility to asthma, as the concordance of asthma in monozygotic twins is much greater than in dizygotic twins. The concordance in monozygotic twins is, however, low, strongly suggesting that environmental factors make important contributions to the development of asthma.

■ Thus not everybody who carries the genes for bronchial hyperreactivity or atopic asthma goes on to develop asthma in childhood or even in later life. It appears that there are critical periods when those with the genetic predisposition are exposed to environmental triggers and go on to develop asthma: the intrauterine period and the first two years of life appear to be the most critical, but occupational asthma may develop in the first two years of exposure to new allergens, even in adulthood.

■ Smoking during pregnancy increases the likelihood of the genetically predisposed baby to develop asthma later on. Smoking during pregnancy also leads to babies with smaller airways and increased cord blood IgE levels. Maternal smoking during the neonatal years may help to increase the sensitization of the child's lungs to other allergens, and increase the risk of developing asthma. Breast-feeding may reduce the chances of a susceptible baby from developing asthma, although the beneficial effects specific for reducing the risk of asthma are less clear than was once thought.

■ If a child has one parent who has atopic asthma, the chance of the child developing asthma in his or her lifetime is about 33%. The chance increases to about 66% if both parents have atopic asthma. Having a sibling with atopic asthma (or other manifestations of atopy) will further increase the likelihood of that child developing asthma. A history of asthma or atopy in more distant relatives is less important, the importance being in proportion to the genetic closeness of the relatives involved.

1.38 At what age does asthma start?

Asthma may occur at any age but usually begins in childhood. Most patients present with symptoms before the age of 2 years, although the diagnosis may not be formally made for some time later. The incidence of new cases peaks by the age of 5 years, may show a slight increase again in the mid-teenage years, and then peaks again for people aged 40–50 years and declines steadily thereafter.

1.39 Is asthma more common in certain races?

Asthma occurs in all races and in all environments. Asthma does not show particularly high or low prevalence rates in any race, with the exceptions of Maoris, who have a higher than expected prevalence, and Australian Aborigines, who have a lower one. There are certainly major differences in the perception of asthma, attitudes towards it, and expectations from management in people from different ethnic groups. This is shown most clearly in the relatively high exacerbation and mortality rates from asthma in UK Asians and in New York blacks and Hispanics.

1.40 Is there a sex bias for asthma?

Atopy occurs more commonly in boys; boys have a smaller airway calibre at birth, so it is not surprising to find that asthma symptoms occur more commonly in boys than in girls. The male preponderance of childhood asthma changes to a female preponderance during adolescence. Asthma presenting in middle age occurs slightly more often in women than in men. Overall, roughly equal numbers of males and females are affected.

1.41 Can we predict whether a newborn baby will become asthmatic?

A careful family history will help to predict the statistical chance of a baby later developing atopic diseases (see Q. 1.45). A raised level of IgE in the cord blood is a highly specific but not very sensitive predictor of subsequent allergic diseases: most babies with a raised cord IgE level will show manifestations of allergic diseases within the first 3 years of life; however, most children who later develop allergy will have had a normal cord IgE level at birth. Measuring the cord blood IgE level is not that helpful.

Intrauterine sensitization to allergens is probably virtually universal, and occurs after about 22 weeks' gestation. The sensitization can be demonstrated by the presence of specific sensitized lymphocytes. Whether this sensitization is of any ultimate importance, or whether demonstrating the presence of these specific lymphocytes will help to predict the later development of allergies, is not known. If it was possible to predict the association between *in utero* exposure to specific allergens at specific gestational ages, a strategy for the primary prevention of asthma might be possible.

1.42 Do premature babies have an increased risk of developing asthma?

Chronic lung disease is common among very premature babies, increasing numbers of whom are surviving into childhood. Most of these children will have recurrent and troublesome respiratory symptoms, including wheezing and night coughs. Their symptoms are likely to continue throughout childhood and, even at 15 years of age, 50% of children who had chronic lung disease secondary to the complications of prematurity will still have evidence of airway obstruction. Many of these children will have asthma, and prematurity (especially if associated with more severe hyaline membrane disease) increases the risks of developing asthma. Children with chronic lung disease respond to bronchodilators, but any decision to use long-term inhaled steroids should be taken only after consultation with the child's hospital team as there may be confounding diagnoses such as tracheal stenosis, bronchopulmonary dysplasia or diaphragm disorders.

MECHANISM OF ASTHMA

1.43 What is the pathology of asthma?

The mechanism of allergic asthma is far better understood than that of non-allergic asthma. Allergic asthma involves three components:

■ Oversensitive lining of the lungs
■ Allergens that trigger the asthmatic allergic response
■ The inflammatory response that occurs as a result of the combination of sensitive lung lining and allergen.

Allergens of a critical particle size of between 1 and 15 microns can escape the upper airway defence mechanism of the body and are large enough to deposit on the walls of small to medium-sized bronchi. The allergens then react with local inflammatory cells.

The *inflammatory allergic response* consists of constriction of the smooth muscle in the bronchi, mucus secretion, fluid leakage from the capillaries and oedema of the bronchial wall. The mucosa of the bronchial walls becomes thickened, inflamed and oedematous. The bronchoconstriction causes the mucosa to pucker and infold, facilitating mucous plugging and airway obstruction (*Fig. 1.12*). The combination of oedema and bronchoconstriction results in narrowing of the bronchi and a marked reduction of airflow through the bronchi. The flow through a tube is

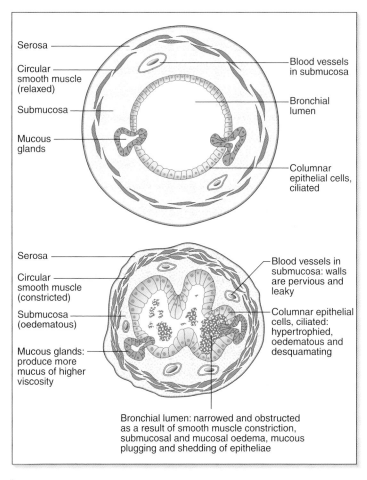

Fig. 1.12 Effects of asthma on the architecture of a bronchiole. *Top*: Bronchiole from a non-asthmatic person or a well-controlled asthmatic. *Bottom*: Bronchiole from a poorly controlled asthmatic.

roughly proportional to the fourth power of the radius of that tube. Thus, if the bronchial radius is halved because of a mixture of inflammation, smooth muscle contraction and swelling of the bronchial mucosa, the flow through the bronchus may be only one-sixteenth of its previous value. Thus small changes in the diameter of the airways have drastic implications on the flow through those airways.

The mechanism of asthma is summarized in *Fig. 1.13*.

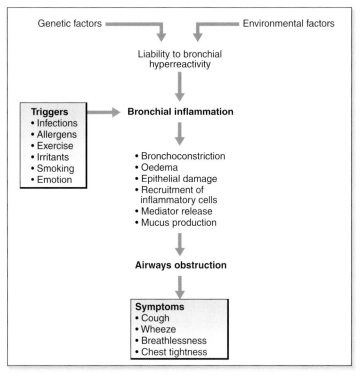

▲

Fig. 1.13 The mechanism of asthma.

1.44 What is the role of inflammation?

Airway inflammation is central to the pathogenesis of all types of asthma. The continued presence of activated eosinophils and mast cells in the lumen and walls of the airways has been demonstrated in many studies, even in patients with supposed mild or asymptomatic asthma. The presence and survival of these inflammatory cells is promoted by the presence of pro-inflammatory cytokines (such as granulocyte–macrophage colony-stimulating factor) in asthmatic airways. The inflammatory cells have the capacity to release mediators such as cysteinyl leukotrienes, which are potent bronchoconstrictors, and which contribute to the airway narrowing in asthma, and for allergen-induced asthma. The inflammatory cascade is also maintained by Th2 lymphocytes. The persisting inflammation, especially airway epithelial damage and altered smooth muscle function, produces airway structural changes, which in turn lead to long-standing hyperresponsiveness of the airways. Mediators such as histamine, thromboxane, platelet-activating factor, leukotrienes and cytokines are released from inflammatory cells and contribute to the chronic airway structural changes.

The precise sequence of events that leads to the presence of persisting airway inflammatory cells, airway structural changes and airway hyperresponsiveness is still not entirely clear.

1.45   Does it matter at what age sensitization and allergen exposure occur?

In uterine life, a significant proportion of fetuses will have a genetic predisposition to atopy. Of these fetuses, only a proportion will actually develop any significant manifestations of allergy. In utero exposure to tobacco smoke and cats will increase the likelihood of a genetically susceptible baby to develop atopy in infancy or in later life, as will exposure to high allergen loads at times of greatest immunological development (from about 3 to 18 months of age, at around 4–4.5 years of age, and in early teenage life). Exposure to certain allergens at these times will further increase the likelihood of developing atopic features. Important allergens include pollens, animal dander (especially cats), cockroaches and house dust mites. There also seems to be some protection against the sensitization from allergens in children who come from large families, or have pet dogs, or have had multiple respiratory infections in childhood. The protection may be related to poor hygiene and therefore a greater exposure of these children to multiple antigens. As a result of the exposure to external antigens, the response of the T lymphocytes is switched from Th2 subtypes to Th1, and therefore away from the production of the Th2 cells that are associated with the development of allergy. (*See Q. 1.30 and Q. 1.32.*)

1.46   What is the effect of the airway inflammation?

A stimulus or exposure to certain triggers will result in inflammation of the susceptible bronchi and bronchioles. This inflammation is more marked in certain individuals who have oversensitive or hyperreactive bronchi. The inflammation may worsen the hyperreactivity. The stimulus or trigger will also cause stimulation of the hyperreactive bronchi directly, which in turn will increase any inflammatory response. The inflammation will lead to epithelial damage, mucosal oedema and mucous plugging; the hyperreactivity will lead to bronchial muscle spasm. The net result is narrowing and obstruction of the small and medium-sized airways, and the symptoms of asthma. If the asthma is persistent and undertreated, the smooth muscle will eventually hypertrophy and irreversible anatomical changes will occur in the small airways.

1.47 Is the inflammation transient or persistent?

It is becoming increasingly clear that in most asthmatics the inflammation is persistent even in the absence of symptoms. This means that managing asthma only by symptom control may lead to persistent, unopposed inflammation in the lungs, which in turn will lead to irreversible anatomical changes and decline in lung function. Early and sustained treatment with anti-inflammatory therapy should therefore be at the forefront of all asthma therapy regimens.

1.48 What happens in non-allergic asthma?

The mechanism of non-allergic asthma is less well understood. The process probably involves stimulation of specific receptors on susceptible individuals' lungs by triggers such as cold air or non-specific irritants, resulting in bronchospasm and bronchial hyperreactivity without allergic airway inflammation.

PQ PATIENT QUESTIONS

1.49 What is asthma?

Asthma is a disease in which there is a reaction of the lining of the lungs. This causes the lining to swell up and become inflamed, and to make the muscles in the small tubes of the lungs more twitchy. The twitchy muscles may tighten and go into spasm in certain situations, or after exposure to various substances, causing narrowing of the tubes. The narrowing results in the symptoms of cough, wheeze, breathlessness and chest tightness.

1.50 Is asthma very common?

Yes, asthma is one of the commonest chronic diseases in the world. About one-fifth of all children in the UK may have asthma at some time, and about one-tenth of adults. The severity of the asthma varies widely between individuals and also in the same person over time. Cases of asthma have doubled in the last ten years in the UK. Asthma has become much more common in many countries of the world, especially in northern and western Europe, North America and Australasia, and also in more affluent city dwellers in developing and tropical countries.

1.51 Why is asthma becoming more common?

No one knows for sure, but there is a variety of factors associated with the increase in asthma over the past 10–15 years, including environmental reasons such as increased levels of house dust mites as our homes become better insulated, pets (especially cats), dusts at work, agricultural changes leading to different and increased pollen loads and cooking with gas. Other factors include changes in diet, improved domestic hygiene and smaller families.

1.52 Does pollution cause asthma?

Probably not, although some forms of pollution can make asthma worse. Although many people think that pollution causes asthma, and that higher pollution levels will cause more and more severe asthma, in fact there is little evidence to support this theory – despite the theory being accepted (erroneously) as fact by the media. For instance, the highest rates of asthma in the UK occur in the highlands and islands of Scotland, and the highest rates in the world occur in New Zealand. Neither of these places is renowned for industrialization or heavy traffic pollution. People living near factories or main roads are actually less likely to develop asthma than those living in the country or suburban areas.

1.53 Can you catch asthma?

No, asthma is not due to any external agent that can be transmitted. Asthma may occur more commonly in families because they share the same genetic predeposition to developing the condition and they are exposed to the same irritants and triggers, such as house dust, pollens and tobacco smoke.

PQ PATIENT QUESTIONS

1.54 Can asthma be cured?

Sadly, no. However, nearly all people with asthma can lead normal lives untroubled by their asthma. Modern management aims to control the disease completely, so the patient has no or very infrequent symptoms, can lead a totally normal life, and have confidence in their long-term asthma control.

1.55 If I have asthma, will my baby develop it too?

Perhaps. There is no single gene for asthma so you will not directly 'pass your asthma on' to your baby. However, there is a strong genetic component to asthma, as it commonly runs in families. If one parent has asthma, there is about a one in three chance of your child developing asthma during his or her lifetime. If both parents are asthmatic, this chance increases to two in three.

Diagnosis of asthma

2

CLINICAL FEATURES

2.1	What are the usual symptoms of asthma?	40
2.2	Does an individual asthmatic patient always have the same symptoms?	40
2.3	What are the usual symptoms in infants and pre-school children?	41
2.4	What are the usual symptoms in adults?	41
2.5	Are symptoms the same in the elderly?	41
2.6	What causes the symptoms of asthma?	41
2.7	Are any symptoms more significant than others?	42
2.8	What are the symptoms of acute severe asthma?	42
2.9	Can you tell what type of asthma a patient has just from the symptoms?	43
2.10	What physical signs can you find in asthmatic patients who are apparently well controlled?	43
2.11	What physical signs can you find in asthmatic patients who are poorly controlled?	43
2.12	What physical signs can you find in patients with acute severe asthma?	43
2.13	Many of the symptoms and signs do not seem specific for asthma. How can you tell clinically that the patient has asthma?	44
2.14	Are there any symptoms and signs that might suggest alternative diagnoses?	44

TESTS AND INVESTIGATIONS

2.15	What tests are most useful in diagnosing asthma?	45
2.16	What about tests in young children and babies?	47
2.17	Are peak flow measurements sufficient or are spirometry readings necessary?	47
2.18	Are all peak flow meters interchangeable?	50
2.19	When should a chest X-ray be ordered?	50
2.20	Are skin prick tests useful or necessary?	51
2.21	Are there any blood tests that are helpful or essential?	51

2.22 Which patients should be referred to a specialist for confirmation of the diagnosis of asthma? 52

2.23 What about gene testing? 52

2.24 Are there any other allergy tests available to patients? 52

2.25 What tests would be most useful in an ideal world? 53

DIFFERENTIAL DIAGNOSIS

2.26 What are the main differential diagnoses at each stage of life? 53

2.27 What are the other manifestations of atopy? 55

2.28 Is asthma associated with otitis media or any other disorders? 55

ASTHMA IN CHILDREN

2.29 How can asthma be confidently diagnosed in pre-school children? 55

2.30 Do all children who cough and wheeze have asthma? 56

2.31 Is there such a condition as wheezy bronchitis? 56

2.32 Do children really grow out of asthma? 56

2.33 Are there any risk factors for childhood asthma that persist into adulthood? 58

2.34 Is there any medical intervention that will reduce the risk of childhood asthma continuing in adulthood? 58

2.35 Does it matter if asthma is overdiagnosed or underdiagnosed, particularly in children? 58

ASTHMA IN ADULTS

2.36 How can asthma be confidently diagnosed in adults? 59

2.37 What about the elderly – can they develop asthma for the first time? 59

2.38 Why does asthma develop in adults? 60

2.39 What is the difference between asthma and chronic obstructive pulmonary disease (COPD)? 61

2.40 Is it important to distinguish between asthma and COPD? 61

ASTHMA AND COMPLICATING FACTORS

2.41 Are there any complications from asthma? 62

2.42 Does smoking make any difference to the way asthma presents or is managed? 62

PATIENT QUESTIONS

2.43 How do I know I've got asthma?   63

2.44 How do I know my child has asthma?   63

2.45 Why do many people seem to have asthma and hay fever
and eczema?   63

2.46 Will my child grow out of the asthma?   63

CLINICAL FEATURES

2.1 What are the usual symptoms of asthma?

Asthma is a very heterogeneous disease, especially in its presentation and severity. As it is a disease characterized by reversible airway narrowing, the clinical features of asthma show great variability both between asthmatics and in the same individual over time. However, the primary problems are the sensitive bronchial mucosa and hyperreactive bronchial muscle, causing bronchial mucosal oedema, increased mucus production and smooth muscle spasm, which lead to airway narrowing (*see Q. 1.43*). This causes the four main symptoms of asthma:

■ Cough
■ Wheeze
■ Shortness of breath
■ Chest tightness.

Bear in mind that patients can present with any combination of these symptoms.

2.2 Does an individual asthmatic patient always have the same symptoms?

One of the characteristic features of asthma is the variability of airflow obstruction and of subsequent symptoms that occur over time, or in response to trigger exposure, or to changes in treatment.

In poorly controlled asthma, symptoms will typically worsen over days or weeks, especially if provoked by triggers such as a cold or change in indoor environment. Symptoms will improve spontaneously or, more usually, in response to treatment, and will return to the same level as before the deterioration, or may even be improved if the resulting treatment is more effective. Recovery usually takes about the same time as it took the patient to develop the most severe symptoms, but can be quicker, and the patient may be back to their best within hours or days.

In patients with more severe asthma, symptoms may worsen much more quickly, often over hours or even within 15–30 minutes of provocation. The provoking agent may not always be apparent or identifiable. Recovery may be slower, or sometimes as rapid as the deterioration.

Patients with mild to moderate asthma will be well, with no symptoms at all between exacerbations. Patients with more severe asthma may never be free of all asthma symptoms, typically having some shortness of breath and wheezing on exertion, and occasional night cough, even when on maximum treatment.

2.3 What are the usual symptoms in infants and pre-school children?

The symptoms can include cough and wheezing, especially with or after an upper respiratory tract infection. A persistent cough, especially at night or after a cold, is common. Persistent or paroxysmal cough, especially if nocturnal, for more than 10–14 days, or following a cold, is likely to be due to asthma and, if recurrent, should be considered as such until proved otherwise.

There may be a history of repeated wheeze, again often at night. Childhood wheezing is significantly associated with prematurity. This association is proportional to the degree of prematurity.

The symptoms are often precipitated by viral infection, exercise or excitement, allergens such as pets or dusts, cigarette smoke or emotional disturbances. Some children are just slightly listless or non-specifically below par.

Small children do not usually complain of chest tightness or feeling short of breath. They may, however, complain of tummy aches or pains, and observers may notice coughing on exertion or an inability of the child to keep up with his or her peers in normal children's activities. Sputum production is rare in small children with asthma.

2.4 What are the usual symptoms in adults?

The characteristic symptoms are paroxysmal wheezing and breathlessness, especially on exertion or after exposure to triggers.

The severity of the symptoms varies greatly. Symptoms may be preceded or accompanied by chest tightness and coughing. Coughing, especially at night or on exertion, may be the predominant feature. Occasionally the cough may be productive of clear, green or yellow sputum, which is usually a product of inflammation of the airways rather than infection.

2.5 Are symptoms the same in the elderly?

Exertional symptoms may not be apparent if patients' ability to exert themselves is limited by other conditions such as osteoarthrosis or cardiac conditions. Many of the symptoms are not specific for asthma and can be overlooked or attributed to concomitant disorders such as heart disease.

2.6 What causes the symptoms of asthma?

Remember that asthma is a chronic inflammatory disease of the airways causing paroxysmal bronchospasm and airway obstruction. The symptoms of asthma are largely due to the resultant airway obstruction. The airway inflammation may not cause any symptoms whatsoever, as the inflammation itself does not necessarily cause significant airway obstruction.

The symptoms of asthma are due to irritation and obstruction of (especially) the small to medium-sized bronchi, secondary to the inflammatory response occurring in the mucosa of the airways from the trachea to the terminal bronchioles.

Shortness of breath and wheeze are due to obstruction of the bronchi caused partly by inflammation and mucosal oedema but mainly by the bronchospasm secondary to that inflammation. Cough and chest tightness are caused by mucosal inflammation and bronchospasm, and by irritation of receptors in the lungs and chest walls.

2.7   Are any symptoms more significant than others?

Not particularly.

- Cough-variant asthma is quite common, especially in children. Cough is the predominant or only symptom, and is usually worse at night or on exertion.
- The severity of wheezing together with the severity of breathlessness reflects the severity of asthma more than the amount of coughing.
- Chest tightness is rarely the only symptom, and is more characteristic of angina.
- Severe shortness of breath is unusual without there being some accompanying wheezing and chest tightness.
- Symptoms that improve with exercise are unlikely to be due to asthma.
- Symptoms that are worse at night or in the early morning, that are recurrent and variable, are characteristic of asthma.
- Worsening of the symptoms in the presence of common triggers, such as pollens, exercise, viral infections and weather changes, is strongly suggestive of asthma.
- A personal or family history of asthma or other atopic manifestation makes the diagnosis of asthma more likely.
- It is unusual for patients to have marked daytime symptoms, but none at night.

2.8   What are the symptoms of acute severe asthma?

- Shortness of breath, especially if the patient cannot talk in sentences or complete activities requiring minimal exertion such as eating, dressing or even walking a few paces.
- Wheezing and chest tightness may be severe.
- Cough may be distressing and debilitating.
- Exhaustion, thirst and feeling dry, vomiting (especially in small children).

2.9 Can you tell what type of asthma a patient has just from the symptoms?

The symptoms will not help distinguish between extrinsic and intrinsic asthma. A good history of what seems to provoke those symptoms may well do so.

2.10 What physical signs can you find in asthmatic patients who are apparently well controlled?

Between exacerbations there are usually no abnormal findings at all. However, it is important to examine all patients with asthma at the initial presentation (even if asymptomatic on that day) to exclude other possible causes of symptoms such as cardiac conditions, anaemia, upper respiratory tract conditions or other lung diseases.

Physical signs of atopic manifestations such as nasal polyps or atopic dermatitis may help in diagnosing asthma. Oedema, chest crackles and clubbing are not features of asthma.

2.11 What physical signs can you find in asthmatic patients who are poorly controlled?

If control has been poor for months or years, there may be chest wall changes (pectus carinatum and Harrison's sulci), especially in children. In adults the chest may be hyperinflated. Such changes are becoming rarer as many more patients have received better and more effective care over the past two or three decades.

2.12 What physical signs can you find in patients with acute severe asthma?

■ Physical signs during a severe acute exacerbation may include audible wheezing, tachycardia, tachypnoea, intercostal recession, and the use of accessory muscles for breathing, distress and even cyanosis. Inability to talk in complete sentences is a sign of a severe attack. Chest auscultation will reveal an overexpanded chest with wheezing or, if very severe, a nearly silent chest.

■ Patients may be dehydrated or exhausted.

■ The global assessment, especially of respiratory rate, cyanosis, exhaustion and distress, are more important than the degree of wheezing.

■ Measuring pulsus paradoxicus is not helpful: it is an unreliable, non-specific sign that may delay the instigation of treatment while not helping with the diagnosis of asthma or in assessing its severity.

2.13 Many of the symptoms and signs do not seem specific for asthma. How can you tell clinically that the patient has asthma?

■ *Symptoms*: The characteristic symptoms of asthma are those of cough, wheeze, chest tightness and shortness of breath, which can occur in any combination, vary in severity over days to weeks, may go completely when the patient is well, and respond completely or at least in part to treatment. Symptoms are usually worse on exertion, and may occur at night.

■ *Family history*: There is often a history of first-degree relatives (parents or siblings) with asthma or other atopic diseases. A family history in more distant relatives is less significant.

■ *Past medical history*: Patients with atopic asthma often have other manifestations of atopy, especially allergic rhinitis, dermatitis or conjunctivitis.

■ *Allergies*: Patients often volunteer allergic reactions to specific triggers, especially pollens, cats, horses or dogs.

■ *Response to treatment*: A clear history of the beneficial effects of bronchodilators (and perhaps of oral steroids), especially if repeated, is diagnostic of asthma. There is no other condition that consistently and significantly responds to the treatments used for asthma.

2.14 Are there any symptoms and signs that might suggest alternative diagnoses?

■ New symptoms of abrupt onset especially in small children suggest an inhaled foreign body.

■ Focal wheezes on auscultation, or fixed crackles or wheezes or crepitations, all suggest alternative reasons for the patient's symptoms.

■ Chest pain, focal chest or chest wall pain or flitting pains are not typical of asthma.

■ Asthma does not cause fever, weight loss, lymphadenopathy, clubbing, haemoptysis or night sweats.

■ Shortness of breath, mainly on exertion, that is of gradual, insidious onset, and is not markedly bad at night, in patients with a history of cigarette smoking for at least 20 years suggests chronic obstructive pulmonary disease (COPD).

■ Breathlessness on bending forward is more usually a feature of COPD than of asthma.

TESTS AND INVESTIGATIONS

2.15 What tests are most useful in diagnosing asthma?

The most useful test is to determine the peak flow. Peak flow meters are cheap, portable and readily available, and their technique is easy to learn and teach. The use of a peak flow meter is shown in *Fig. 2.1*.

Peak flow readings that vary by 20% or more, either spontaneously or in response to treatment, are diagnostic of asthma. There are no other conditions in which peak flow readings will show this amount of variability.

Serial readings, over time and in response to therapy, are needed. Twice-daily peak flow charts, with readings taken as soon as possible after waking and at about 6pm, will demonstrate any diurnal variation as well as providing baseline readings. Children from the age of 5–6 years, and most adults, are capable of using peak flow measurements. Patients need to be taught how to use the meter properly. Three readings are normally taken, and the best of the three is the one that is recorded.

The peak flow is expressed as litres per minute (L/min) and normal ranges vary with age, sex and height. The reading will be decreased in proportion to the severity of the airway obstruction. A peak flow chart from a previously undiagnosed asthmatic is shown in *Fig. 2.2*.

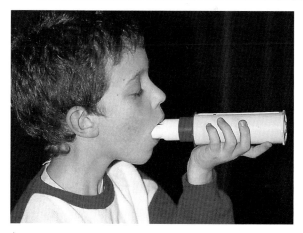

▲

Fig. 2.1 Peak flow meter. This device is easy to use and cheap. Serial readings are invaluable for diagnosing asthma and for assessing the severity of exacerbations and response to any interventions. From Lissauer T (2001), *Illustrated Textbook of Paediatrics* 2nd edn. Edinburgh: Mosby.

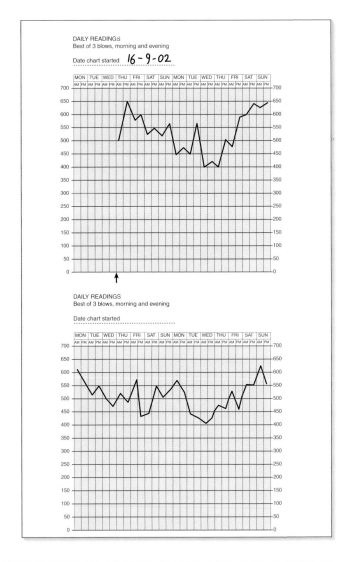

Fig. 2.2 Serial peak flow readings from a previously undiagnosed asthmatic. The readings demonstrate variability of more than 25%, with marked diurnal variation; the best readings are those predicted for someone of this man's age and height. The variability in the peak flow readings, together with reversibility of the readings to expected normal levels, are diagnostic of asthma. Predicted peak flow in a male caucasian aged 46 years is 645 litres per minute.

The peak flow readings of non-asthmatic subjects show very little variability; there is a small reduction in peak flows when the person has a cold and only minor increases in peak flow in response to bronchodilators.

Exercise tests may also be useful. The patient takes a peak flow reading, then exercises to breathlessness. Serial peak flow readings are then taken at 5-minute intervals for 30 minutes. Again, a fall in the peak flow values of 20% or more is significant and diagnostic of exercise-provoked asthma.

In patients with peak flows below the expected levels, reversibility testing may be diagnostic if the therapy used results in an improvement in the peak flow reading of 20% or more. The usual therapy is inhaled bronchodilator, administered via a large-volume spacer or a nebulizer, and the post-bronchodilator readings should be taken 15–20 minutes after administration of the therapy. If the result is still equivocal, a trial of oral steroids for 2–3 weeks at a dose of 1–2 mg/kg bodyweight is the gold standard. An improvement in peak flow readings of 20% or more confirms the diagnosis of asthma, irrespective of any changes in symptoms, as shown in *Fig. 2.3*.

Patients whose initial peak flow readings are at least 20% below the expected readings, and whose readings show no improvement with inhaled bronchodilator or oral steroid therapy, have irreversible obstructive airway disease. They do not have asthma and will not benefit from asthma treatment.

Patients who show a response of less than 20% have partially reversible or mixed obstructive airway disease and may respond to asthma treatment.

A diagnostic algorithm for the diagnosis of asthma is shown in *Fig. 2.4*.

2.16   What about tests in young children and babies?

Children under the age of 6–7 years cannot reliably and consistently use a peak flow meter. There are no other tests of airway function and reversibility available, so in practice a diagnosis of asthma in babies and young children is made entirely on the history and on the response of the child to treatment. Abolition of symptoms by using regular preventive therapy, or a rapid resolution of symptoms with relieving therapy, is usually diagnostic, especially if the response can be reproduced on one or more occasions.

2.17   Are peak flow measurements sufficient or are spirometry readings necessary?

Airway obstruction can be documented most reliably by means of the forced expiratory volume in 1 second (FEV_1). A spirometer is needed to measure FEV_1; reliable and portable spirometers are available and are becoming more widely used in general practice. Airway obstruction is defined as an FEV_1 that is lower than the predicted value minus 840 mL in men and 620 mL in women. The best method of assessing reversibility in

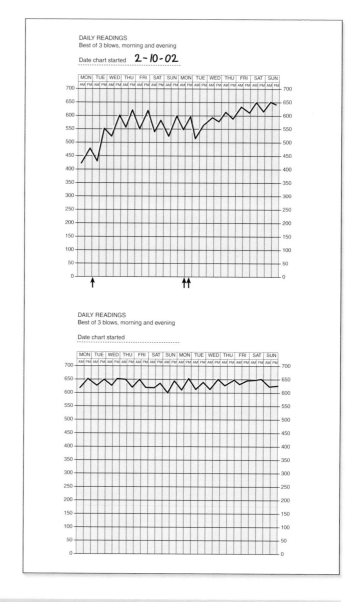

Fig. 2.3 Serial peak flow readings from the same patient as in *Fig. 2.2*, showing responses to: (a) regular inhaled short-acting β₂-agonists (↑) and (b) the addition of regular inhaled steroids (↑↑).

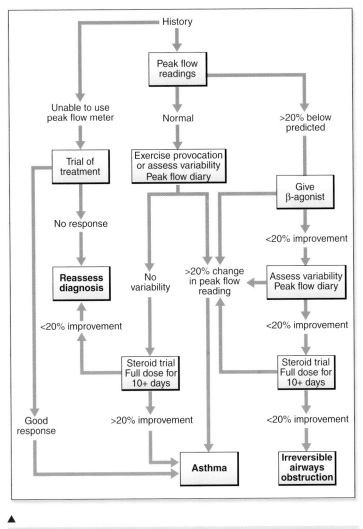

Fig. 2.4 The diagnosis of asthma.

airway obstruction using a spirometer is by expressing the change in FEV_1 as a percentage of the predicted value. A change in FEV_1 of 20% or more of the predicted value indicates reversibility. Reversibility of airway obstruction is determined by the same method used when assessing peak flow changes.

Peak flow meter assessment is not quite as accurate as a FEV_1 measurement in determining the severity of airway obstruction. However, peak flow meters are as effective in determining reversibility and variability of airway obstruction in patients with asthma. Peak flow measurements are simple and reproducible, and offer a quantitative assessment of airway resistance or obstruction. Peak flow meters are much cheaper and easier to use than spirometers, and are the device of choice for the diagnosis and assessment of nearly all asthmatics managed in primary care.

The peak flow meter does not show good long-term correlation with FEV_1. Some patients with severe asthma and all patients with COPD will show a long-term decline in lung function. This will be detected by serial measurements of FEV_1 but not of peak flow.

2.18 Are all peak flow meters interchangeable?

Standard-range meters (60–800 L/min) are suitable for most adults and older children; low-range meters (40–350 L/min) are best used by children aged 5 years or over, or by adults with consistently low flows (it helps their morale).

It is sensible for general practitioners to prescribe the same meter that they use in their surgeries. It is also important to appreciate that different makes of meter are not entirely compatible. Changes in peak flow are best assessed when the same meter is used consistently with the same patient. The meters may over-read by up to 80 L/min at the middle ranges. This may lead to slight underestimation of the peak flow and to undertreatment, although whether this has any clinical implications remains unproven.

Most of the commonly used mzst for about 3 years. Peak flow readings should be taken on waking, before going to bed, and on at least two other occasions each day for which recordings are requested. Readings should always be taken before any bronchodilator is used. Every asthmatic should know their best-ever or predicted levels. They should also have their use of the meter and ability to read and record their readings checked by their doctor or nurse at least annually.

2.19 When should a chest X-ray be ordered?

- When the history suggests an inhaled foreign body, or if there are symptoms or signs that are not typical of asthma, or in a patient with asthma who is deteriorating despite maximum therapy.
- A chest X-ray is also advisable on the first presentation of middle-aged or elderly patients with symptoms suggestive of asthma but who smoke or who used to smoke.
- When there is a possibility of pneumonia or bronchiolitis, especially if the patient is unwell or toxic.

■ A chest X-ray is also recommended in patients with an occupational history of asbestos, coal dust, metal or mineral exposure.

■ If there is any doubt that the patient may be at risk of tuberculosis.

2.20 Are skin prick tests useful or necessary?

Skin prick tests can be used to help identify whether a patient is likely to be sensitive to specific allergens. The tests are available for a large range of potential allergens.

The test kits are relatively cheap (about £100) and need to be kept in a fridge. They are not reimbursable, nor are they available on prescription. Although severe allergic reactions are very rare, it is advisable to have available facilities and equipment for resuscitation when skin prick-testing patients.

They can be used to identify or confirm an allergic tendency to specific allergens. However, a positive skin prick test result does not prove that the patient is definitely allergic to that potential allergen, and neither does a negative test rule out the patient being sensitive to that potential allergen. A positive test result in an atopic individual will not differentiate the severity or type of reaction of that individual to exposure to that allergen. The reaction may show as atopic dermatitis, allergic rhinitis or conjunctivitis, or as asthma – or as any combination.

Skin prick test results are unreliable in patients taking antihistamines or antidepressants, and in the elderly or very young.

Their use should be considered in patients who reasonably request testing, or in patients who might be allergic to specific allergens and are willing and able to take action to avoid future allergen exposure. Examples include an atopic child whose parents ask whether they could get a cat, or to help parents decide whether anti-house dust mite measures are worth considering.

In practice, skin prick test results are not always very useful in managing asthma, as the tests are often positive to allergens that the patient cannot – or chooses not – to avoid. *See also Q. 4.6.*

2.21 Are there any blood tests that are helpful or essential?

Blood tests are not usually very helpful. The eosinophil count in the peripheral blood film may be raised in atopic disorders, but a normal eosinophil level does not rule out atopy. The level of eosinophilia is not a good marker of the severity of an individual's asthma.

Serum immunoglobulin (Ig) E levels may also be increased in some patients with asthma, but again the levels are not diagnostic and do not correlate with the severity of asthma.

Radioallergosorbent (RAST) tests may be used to identify or confirm allergy to specific allergens, such as house dust mite, cats, horses or

Aspergillus. More than 450 specific allergen tests are available. In practice, these tests are most useful in refractory asthma or in diagnosing aspergillosis, but otherwise are usually more useful in people with food or drug allergies and dermatitis, or where skin prick tests are unreliable, as detailed in Q. 2.24

2.22 Which patients should be referred to a specialist for confirmation of the diagnosis of asthma?

■ Patients who do not respond to conventional therapy in a predicted fashion, or those whose response is not as complete as expected.
■ Patients who have concomitant diseases, such as cardiac failure, ischaemic heart disease, asbestosis or pulmonary tuberculosis.
■ The younger the baby with possible asthma, the lower the threshold for referral for confirmation of the diagnosis should be. This is especially true if the baby was born prematurely or had any neonatal respiratory problems.
■ Patients with possible mixed obstructive airway disease (smokers or ex-smokers in middle or old age), especially if the primary care team does not have access to a spirometer.

2.23 What about gene testing?

There are many genes associated with atopy and asthma. At present it is not feasible to perform intrauterine fetal blood sampling or amniotic fluid cytology to ascertain the genetic status of the fetus. If techniques were developed to allow such tests to be safely performed, the knowledge gained would be of value in only a few cases. It would be unethical and undesirable to consider aborting babies at risk of developing asthma. There are no completely proven interventions applicable to a fetus with a genetic status compatible with a high risk of later developing asthma. Strategies that may be advocated are much the same as those currently advocated for at-risk babies, or for babies born with high cord blood levels of IgE: no maternal smoking in pregnancy, no exposure of the baby to tobacco smoke in the first few years of life, minimal allergen exposure in utero and after birth, and recommendations for the mother to breast-feed.

2.24 Are there any other allergy tests available to patients?

■ *Cord IgE levels*: There is some correlation between high cord blood IgE levels at birth and the later development of asthma. However, the levels are not particularly specific or sensitive.
■ *Internet allergy tests*: There is a variety of allergy tests available privately for patients, not all of which are scientifically based and reliable. The

main drawbacks are that such tests may not be carried out to consistently rigorous standards, may have no proven scientific or clinical basis, and may have low sensitivity and specificity. There does seem to be a tendency for an extraordinary proportion of tests to come back showing 'definite allergy to . . .'.

2.25 What tests would be most useful in an ideal world?

The most useful test would be a reliable, specific and sensitive marker of airway inflammation that could be quickly, easily and reliably measured in the surgery or the patient's home. This would allow a more exact, individualized dose of preventive therapy to be used by each patient, who could vary this dose and that of any relievers according to the varying amounts of airway inflammation occurring in their lungs.

Exhaled levels of nitric oxide (NO) have shown some promise as a marker of bronchial inflammation in some research centres. NO plays an important role as a vasodilator, neurotransmitter and inflammatory mediator. There is some correlation between NO levels and other markers of airway inflammation, but there is no practical way that levels of exhaled NO can be measured, especially in primary care.

Portable spirometers that measure FEV_1 and forced vital capacity (FVC) quickly and reliably, and instantly calculate the predicted levels and percentages of predicted levels obtained from the patient, may be of use for a large number of patients, especially those with unstable asthma.

A blood test or some other marker that would reliably and accurately predict the atopic status of an individual, especially newborn babies or even fetuses, would allow early and accurate diagnosis of asthma.

Quick, cheap, reliable allergy tests that would accurately describe all the major allergens for an individual at risk would be most useful.

DIFFERENTIAL DIAGNOSIS

2.26 What are the main differential diagnoses at each stage of life?

Many small babies and infants may wheeze when they have colds or other respiratory tract infections. Some of these infants have viral induced wheeze, which probably does not involve inflammation of the airways and therefore is unlikely to be true asthma. However, if these infants also have a strong family history of asthma, or any other atopic features, they may well have asthma. This is especially true if they have symptoms between colds or viral infections. The distinction between virus-induced wheeze and infant asthma is difficult and often becomes clear only with the passage of time.

Infection of the small tubes in the lungs is probably the commonest differential diagnosis in babies and small infants. Again the distinction between asthma and bronchiolitis can be very difficult, especially without recourse to chest radiography. Other possible causes of recurrent wheezing in infancy are shown in *Box 2.1*. In older children and adults acute bronchitis can mimic acute asthma. In the elderly, the distinction between COPD (emphysema or chronic bronchitis) and asthma is extremely

---

BOX 2.1 Causes of recurrent wheezing in infants

- Asthma.
- Recurrent viral infections.

These two diagnoses probably account for 70–90% of all cases of recurrent wheeze. Less common causes include:

- Postrespiratory syncitial virus infections (bronchiolitis) – usually a single, prolonged episode.
- Recurrent aspiration of gastric contents – often positional symptoms, worse on lying flat.
- Premature baby – especially if the baby was ventilated.
- Cystic fibrosis – usually with failure to thrive.
- Maternal smoking – causing irritation to the baby's lungs.
- Inhaled foreign body – usually abrupt onset; wheeze may be focal or unilateral.
- Congenital lung, heart or chest wall abnormality – usually additional symptoms and signs.
- Idiopathic.

TABLE 2.1 Differential diagnosis of asthma

Age group	Common	Uncommon
Babies, small infants	Virus-induced wheeze	Inhaled foreign body Bronchiolitis Cystic fibrosis Cardiac failure Whooping cough
School-aged children	Bronchitis Chronic catarrhal rhinitis	
Adults	Chronic obstructive pulmonary disease Chronic catarrhal rhinitis Acute bronchitis Angina or cardiac failure Postnasal drip Lung cancer	Pneumothorax Allergic alveolitis Diffuse pulmonary fibrosis Sarcoidosis

blurred, and often the two affect the same patient. Acute asthma and left ventricular failure may be difficult to diagnose, especially in the elderly.

Other different diagnoses are listed in *Table 2.1*

2.27   What are the other manifestations of atopy?

When the allergic response involves a specific IgE-mediated reaction and is associated with a genetic predisposition to allergies such as asthma, eczema, hay fever and urticaria, the individual is said to be atopic or to have atopy, which is manifested as:

- Atopic asthma
- Atopic dermatitis
- Allergic rhinitis (especially hay fever)
- Allergic conjunctivitis
- Urticaria.

Atopic patients may experience one or more of these atopic manifestations at any one time.

2.28   Is asthma associated with otitis media or any other disorders?

Yes, asthmatics have an increased incidence of secretory otitis media. Other associations with asthma include increased incidences of nasal polyps, recurrent or chronic sinusitis, and other catarrhal illnesses. Successful treatment or control of these associated features often greatly improves asthma control and is occasionally a prerequisite for successful asthma care.

ASTHMA IN CHILDREN

2.29   How can asthma be confidently diagnosed in pre-school children?

In pre-school children, the diagnosis is usually made by:

- Obtaining a good history, especially of persistent night-time cough, of symptoms suggestive of asthma (*see Q. 2.8*), and including a family history of asthma and of atopy.
- An improvement in the child's symptoms as ascertained by the assessment of a parent or carer, in response to relieving treatment.
- This improvement should be on at least two separate occasions.
- Alternatively, there should be improvements in the child's long-term symptoms in response to long-term preventive therapy.
- There are no confirmatory tests available to prove or confirm the diagnosis.

2.30 Do all children who cough and wheeze have asthma?

Not all children with episodic coughing and wheezing will necessarily have asthma. Wheezing and coughing are very common symptoms in children.

- Some children have recurrent coughs or wheezing but no features of atopy, and no family history. These children usually have symptoms only in response to viral infections. They have virus-associated wheeze rather than asthma, and almost certainly do not have any long-term inflammation in the airways.
- Some children have symptoms of possible asthma plus other atopic features or a strong family history of asthma, and have symptoms between upper respiratory tract infections. These children are very likely to have asthma and also to have chronic inflammation of the airways.
- Some children have symptoms of possible asthma plus atopic features or a strong family history of asthma, but have symptoms only or mostly in response to upper respiratory tract infections. These children fall between the two other extremes, and may have asthma. See *Fig. 2.5*.

2.31 Is there such a condition as wheezy bronchitis?

Euphemisms and synonyms for asthma include:

- Wheezy bronchitis
- A bad (or weak) chest
- Prone to colds and coughs
- Catarrh on the chest
- Colds go to the chest.

None of the above terms is particularly helpful or specific, and should not be used. The exception may be 'wheezy bronchitis'. This is a term more widely used in the past but becoming more common recently, which describes children who have elements of bronchiolitis or other chest infections and who have audible wheezing – a mixture of airway infection together with airway obstruction. The term does not imply that the infection is the cause of the obstruction, or vice versa, nor does it necessarily exclude a diagnosis of asthma. It is a useful term because many of these children will require both antibiotic and bronchodilator therapy for the acute episode, and long-term follow-up, as a high proportion will eventually demonstrate symptoms and signs of asthma.

2.32 Do children really grow out of asthma?

The answer must be yes. It is generally accepted that asthma is more prevalent in children than in adults (in the UK, the rates are about 10% and

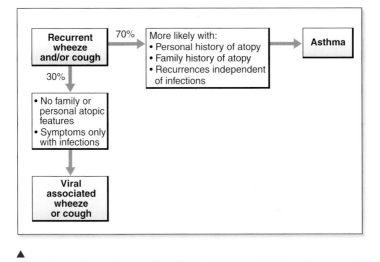

Fig. 2.5 Asthma and virus-associated wheeze.

5% respectively). As asthma can start at any age, it is logical that a large proportion of children who have asthma lose their tendency to have the disease or its symptoms as they grow into adulthood. A number of children will, of course, have been misdiagnosed, and had virus-associated wheeze or other causes for the symptoms. However, it is likely that at least a similar number (which is incalculable) will actually have or have had asthma, but never been formally diagnosed. Simple arithmetic therefore provides the answer that some children must grow out of asthma.

Of 100 children aged 7 years with diagnosed asthma, approximately 25% will be symptom-free and have normal pulmonary function test results at age 20; a further 25% will have persistent, troublesome asthma; and the remaining 50% will have very mild symptoms and small changes in their pulmonary function, especially after provocation by, for example, viral infections. However, 30% of those patients who had childhood asthma but were symptom-free at age 20 will have had re-emergence of their symptoms by the age of 30.

Thus, only about one-third of childhood asthmatics will continue to have asthma on into adulthood. Why the remaining two-thirds undergo remission is not known. The improvement during adolescence may be due to hormonal changes resulting in decreased clinical and immune responsiveness, or the hormonal changes may affect the airways directly, changing the inflammatory response and the smooth muscle and vascular functions.

2.33 Are there any risk factors for childhood asthma that persist into adulthood?

Risk factors of childhood asthma persisting into adulthood include:

■ Female sex
■ Onset before three years of age, especially if frequent symptoms in infancy
■ More than ten acute exacerbations
■ Persistently low peak flow in childhood
■ Parental asthma
■ Continued exposure to allergen.

2.34 Is there any medical intervention that will reduce the risk of childhood asthma continuing in adulthood?

This has exciting possibilities as targeting such individuals for intensive treatment may alter the natural course of disease. Indeed, it has been shown that early treatment with inhaled corticosteroids may actually prevent the development of persistent airway changes. Early treatment with inhaled steroids can certainly produce long-term control of the asthma, which can be maintained on lower doses than would have been needed if the introduction of inhaled steroids had been delayed.

Environmental intervention should also be particularly effective in children who have inherited or acquired characteristics that put them at risk of developing asthma. Reducing the allergen load to babies at high risk of developing asthma (*see Q. 1.41 and Q. 1.45*), both in utero and in the first two years of life, may reduce the chances of that infant developing asthma, or reduce and modify the severity of the asthma should it occur.

2.35 Does it matter if asthma is overdiagnosed or underdiagnosed, particularly in children?

UNDERDIAGNOSIS

Underdiagnosis will lead to undertreatment and poor asthma control. Children will receive inadequate or inappropriate treatment for their symptoms, which will therefore be more severe and prolonged. The child will be denied the benefits of long-term preventive therapy (especially inhaled steroids) and the beneficial effects of such therapy on modifying the chronic inflammation in the airways and of reducing the otherwise permanent airway remodelling. Untreated or poorly treated asthma leads to poor asthma control, prolonged symptoms, airway remodelling and long-term lung damage, and a poorer prognosis. In addition, the parents and carers are more likely to be dissatisfied and disillusioned with their medical care, with poor doctor–patient relationships and worse adherence to future management options.

OVERDIAGNOSIS

Overdiagnosis will lead to overtreatment or unnecessary treatment, which is unlikely to be harmful but is a waste of money on unnecessary medication, and of the patient's, parent's or carer's time. There may be lifestyle changes (such as a decision not to have a dog) decided by the child's family, as well as the psychological burden and worry that comes from a child being diagnosed as having a chronic incurable disease – even if asthma is a disease that is usually easily managed. A misdiagnosis of asthma may mean that other causes of the patient's symptoms (such as cystic fibrosis) may have been overlooked.

ASTHMA IN ADULTS

2.36 How can asthma be confidently diagnosed in adults?

HISTORY

- Cough, wheeze, shortness of breath and chest tightness of variable severity, commonly worse with or after exercise and cold, and which improves over time either in response to treatment or spontaneously. Symptoms may be prominent at night.
- Often an accompanying history of allergic rhinitis and/or atopic dermatitis.
- Often a family history of atopy.

EXAMINATION

- Usually normal between episodes.
- If the patient has more severe asthma, wheezing throughout both lung fields.

TESTS

- Peak flow readings, which will show 20% variability or more over time or in response to therapy. This variability is diagnostic in itself and such readings should always be attempted, if possible, before making a firm diagnosis. No other tests are usually helpful or necessary.

2.37 What about the elderly – can they develop asthma for the first time?

Asthma can start at any age, and asthma in the elderly is not uncommon. The usual symptoms are cough and wheeze, especially on exertion. Many patients will have had symptoms for many years before presentation but have not brought themselves to medical attention as the symptoms may have been wrongly dismissed by the patient as being part of the normal ageing process, or because the patient feared a more sinister diagnosis – or feared dismissal by the doctor.

In patients aged over 40 years, the main differential diagnosis is of COPD, especially in smokers or ex-smokers. This is discussed more fully in *Q. 2.39* and as detailed in *Table 2.2*.

Once a diagnosis has been secured, the management is no different from that for other adults, although particular attention needs to be paid to any potential drug interactions and difficulties with inhaler technique.

2.38 Why does asthma develop in adults?

Asthma that develops in adults is either a re-emergence of symptoms in patients whose childhood asthma has recurred after a period of apparent

TABLE 2.2 Main differences between asthma and chronic obstructive pulmonary disease (COPD)

	COPD	Asthma
History		
Smoker	Nearly always current or ex-smoker	Not relevant
Childhood chest problems	Not usually relevant	Often
Cough and sputum	Common, especially in mornings and as everyday symptoms	Less common, especially as everyday symptoms
Onset of breathlessness	Insidious, gradual	Paroxysmal
Variability of symptoms	Little	Marked
Night symptoms	Uncommon	Common
Symptom mixture	Mainly breathlessness on exertion with persistent cough, often productive; wheeze may develop later	May be none if well; If less well, cough, wheeze, breathlessness and chest tightness can occur together or in any combination
Tests		
PEF and FEV_1	Low	Normal or low
β_2-Agonist response	Little or none	Marked (>20%)
PEF variability	Little or none	More common, especially diurnal
Blood eosinophilia	No	Common
Steroid response	Little or none	Good

PEF, peak expiratory flow; FEV_1, forced expiratory volume in 1 second remission, or is asthma that has developed de novo in adulthood. It is likely that some patients in the latter category should be in the former one, but their childhood symptoms were never properly diagnosed or treated.

Asthma that develops de novo in adulthood is not usually atopic or allergic. Persistent or recurrent environmental, especially occupational, exposure to triggers is important in many cases.

Risk factors for persistence include:

■ Severe asthma
■ Irreversible component
■ Onset over the age of 40 years
■ Negative skin test result
■ Continuous exposure to occupational agents.

2.39 What is the difference between asthma and chronic obstructive pulmonary disease (COPD)?

COPD is a common disease that usually affects middle-aged and elderly patients who smoke or who have smoked at least 20 cigarettes a day for 20 years or more. It is an incurable, invariably progressive, disease that responds poorly to pharmaceutical intervention in comparison to the response of most patients with asthma. The distinguishing features are summarized in *Table 2.2*.

2.40 Is it important to distinguish between asthma and COPD?

Yes, the distinction is important so that the most appropriate therapies can be given. Failure to do so can result in the following scenarios:

MISDIAGNOSING COPD AS ASTHMA

■ Overtreatment with inhaled steroids and undertreatment with β_2-agonists or inhaled anticholinergic drugs.
■ Failure to offer more appropriate therapy for COPD, including consideration of oxygen therapy and pulmonary rehabilitation.

MISDIAGNOSING ASTHMA AS COPD

■ Undertreatment with inhaled steroids (and possible failure to prevent airway remodelling) and overtreatment with β_2-agonists or inhaled anticholinergic drugs.
■ Predictable failure to improve the patient's lung function and achieve complete symptom control.
■ Failure to influence and probably improve the patient's symptom control and long-term stability, and failure to improve the long-term control of the patient's asthma.

LIKELY RESULTS OF MISDIAGNOSING EITHER CONDITION

■ Secondary loss of morale and confidence by patient, carer, family and clinician.

ASTHMA AND COMPLICATING FACTORS

2.41 Are there any complications from asthma?

FROM ACUTE SEVERE ASTHMA

■ Death from hypoxia, exhaustion or dehydration
■ Pneumothorax.

FROM ASTHMA POORLY CONTROLLED IN THE LONG TERM

■ Further poor long-term control
■ Increased rate and severity of acute exacerbations
■ Airway remodelling and subsequent loss of reversibility of airway obstruction

2.42 Does smoking make any difference to the way asthma presents or is managed?

PRESENTATION

Smokers are more prone to recurrent acute bronchitis as well as being at increased risk of COPD. Smokers themselves may regard their recurrent respiratory symptoms as normal. Smokers with asthma thus risk being underdiagnosed and may present late.

MANAGEMENT

There are no major differences in managing asthmatics who do and who do not smoke. Asthmatic smokers should be encouraged to stop at every opportunity. Smoking will increase the airway irritability, mucous gland dysplasia and hyperplasia, and speed up the process of airway remodelling and subsequent development of irreversible airway obstruction.

PQ PATIENT QUESTIONS

2.43 How do I know I've got asthma?

The symptoms of asthma, described above, will come and go depending on your activities and circumstances. The first symptoms are often recurrent cough and wheezing, which may be worse at night, on exertion and in cold air. You may feel short of breath with the cough and wheeze, and also on exercise. The symptoms will come and go, usually lasting for hours or days, and you may feel completely well between these episodes. Colds and other viruses may set off attacks. You may get some chest tightness when the other symptoms are particularly severe. You may often have a family history of asthma, eczema and hay fever, or you may have hay fever or eczema yourself.

2.44 How do I know my child has asthma?

Babies and toddlers can get asthma. They will often have a recurrent cough, usually worse at night, and which often accompanies and follows a cold. There may be some wheezing with the cough. Fever, rashes and colds are not due to asthma. Older children may present with recurrent coughs that are worse at night and on exertion. The diagnosis is not always certain as there is no test that will prove the diagnosis in young children and babies. The pattern of symptoms over time, or the response to different treatments, is often helpful in making the diagnosis of asthma, so sometimes it is not easy or even desirable to make a diagnosis too readily.

2.45 Why do many people seem to have asthma and hay fever and eczema?

All of these conditions occur commonly together or in any combination. The usual underlying cause is atopy – an oversensitive immune system by which susceptible people overreact to exposure to common irritants or allergens.

2.46 Will my child grow out of the asthma?

There are far more children than adults with the diagnosis or symptoms of asthma. Many adults develop asthma in adulthood, so simple arithmetic must lead us to conclude that a large number of children do grow out of their asthma. However, a number of these children will not definitely have had asthma, as the diagnosis cannot always be proven. Many other children will lose the symptoms of asthma but still have a permanent tendency towards asthma, and the disease could become evident later in life. In general, the more severe the child's asthma symptoms and the more secure the diagnosis of asthma, the less likely the child will grow out of the asthma.

Natural history, prognosis and costs of asthma

3

NATURAL HISTORY OF ASTHMA AND PROGNOSIS

3.1	What is the natural history of asthma in children?	66
3.2	Can intervention alter the natural history of asthma in children?	66
3.3	How can we predict which children might have asthma persisting into adulthood?	67
3.4	Are there any risk factors for asthma persisting into adulthood?	67
3.5	What is the natural history of asthma in adults?	68
3.6	What happens to asthmatics whose asthma is well controlled?	69
3.7	What happens to asthmatics whose asthma is poorly controlled?	69

EFFECTS OF ASTHMA

3.8	What effect does having asthma have on patients?	69
3.9	What effect does having asthma have on the parents or carers and families of patients?	70
3.10	How many people die from asthma each year?	71
3.11	Which patients are most at risk of fatal asthma?	72

COSTS AND CONSEQUENCES OF ASTHMA

3.12	What are the costs of asthma to the nation?	73
3.13	Does asthma get worse with age?	75
3.14	Does smoking or occupation affect the prognosis of asthma?	76
3.15	Can asthma cause long-term lung damage?	76
3.16	Do adults lose their asthmatic tendency?	76
3.17	What factors may lead to long-term improvements or deterioration of asthma?	76

NATURAL HISTORY OF ASTHMA AND PROGNOSIS

3.1 What is the natural history of asthma in children?

Only about a third of childhood asthmatics will continue to have asthma on into adulthood (*see Q. 2.32*). Why the remaining two-thirds undergo remission is not known. A number of children may have been misdiagnosed as asthmatic. Any improvement during adolescence may be due to hormonal changes resulting in decreased clinical and immune responsiveness, or the hormonal changes may affect the airways directly, changing the inflammatory response. Of the 30% of childhood asthmatics who have symptoms that persist into adulthood, there are various factors that make an individual more likely to have persistent symptoms (*Box 3.1*).

BOX 3.1 Risk factors of childhood asthma persisting into adulthood

- Female sex
- Age of onset at 2 years or above
- More than ten acute exacerbations
- Persistently low peak flow in childhood
- Parental asthma
- Continued exposure to allergen
- Infantile eczema or rhinitis.

3.2 Can intervention alter the natural history of asthma in children?

This has exciting possibilities as targeting such individuals for intensive treatment may alter the natural course of disease. Indeed it has been shown that early treatment with inhaled corticosteroids may actually prevent development of persistent airway changes. Early treatment with inhaled steroids can certainly produce long-term control of the asthma, which can be maintained on lower doses than would have been needed if the introduction of inhaled steroids had been delayed. There is further evidence that severe attacks and chronic disability in childhood asthma can be reduced by effective treatment, and that early and prolonged use of inhaled steroids leads to improvements in any airway remodelling.[1]

It has been established that the natural rate of decline in lung function with age is accelerated by asthma. Early treatment of asthma with inhaled steroids soon after diagnosis preserves lung function and, if applied to those with more severe disease, the inevitable rate of decline in lung function can be slowed by the addition of inhaled steroids.

It seems logical that delaying the use of anti-inflammatory treatment may result in irreversible airway damage.

Environmental intervention could be particularly effective in children who have inherited or acquired characteristics that put them at risk of developing asthma, but are time consuming and expensive. The necessary interventions needed for each individual at risk need to be researched and implemented (*see also Q. 2.33*).

3.3   How can we predict which children might have asthma persisting into adulthood?

Not all children with episodic coughing and wheezing will necessarily have asthma. Wheezing and coughing are common symptoms at some stage of childhood. It is likely that children with symptoms that could be due to asthma can be divided into three categories:

- Those with symptoms but no features of atopy, and with no family history. These children usually have symptoms only in response to viral infections. These children have virus-associated wheeze and almost certainly do not have any long-term inflammation of the airways. They therefore do not need long-term preventive treatment, although they may need bronchodilators as required with upper respiratory tract infections.
- Those with symptoms plus other atopic features or a strong family history of asthma, and who have symptoms attributable to asthma between upper respiratory tract infections. These children are likely to have asthma and to have chronic inflammation of the airways. They therefore need full preventive treatment with anti-inflammatories.
- Those who have symptoms plus atopic features or strong family history of asthma, but who develop symptoms only or mostly in response to upper respiratory tract infections. These children fall between the two other extremes, and may have asthma. They may have chronic inflammatory airway disease and therefore may need preventive treatment. However, the position is less clear-cut and sometimes a 'wait and see' policy is best (*see also Q. 2.32*).

3.4   Are there any risk factors for asthma persisting into adulthood?

There are some risk factors for persistence:

- Severe asthma
- Irreversible component
- Onset over the age of 40 years
- Negative skin test result
- Continuous exposure to occupational agents.

Some asthmatic adults may merely be experiencing a relapse in their childhood asthma; this is more likely if the individual is atopic and smokes (*see also Q. 2.32*).

In summary, there are certain factors that will help in predicting which asthmatic child may 'grow out of it':

■ If the age of onset is over 10 years, the prognosis is poor.
■ Multiple allergic manifestations are associated with a poorer prognosis.
■ The more severe the symptoms, the worse the prognosis.
■ If close relatives with childhood asthma 'grew out of it', the better the prognosis.

It is sensible to continue follow-up and surveillance for at least two years after the last treatment needed for the last asthmatic symptoms. It is also sensible to point out to patients and parents that symptoms may recur at any time in the future.

In adults and children, one of the most rewarding prospects in treating asthma is the possibility of reducing the long-term lung damage that may occur in badly treated or undertreated asthma by using early and full-dose preventive or protective therapy. Poorly treated asthma may eventually lead to long-term lung damage. The long-term use of inhaled anti-inflammatory agents used to control asthma may help this trend. In children, vigorous treatment of infants at risk of developing asthma with high-dose inhaled steroids at their first presentation might reduce the sensitization and inhibit the subsequent severity or chronicity of asthma.

3.5 What is the natural history of asthma in adults?

Most adults with asthma have also had childhood asthma. Some will have had persistent asthma right through adolescence. Of those who develop asthma as adults, the exact mechanism of the development is unknown. Most asthma that develops in adults who did not have childhood asthma is either non-allergic, or allergic but not atopic. Environmental, especially occupational, exposure to triggers is important in many cases. It may be that some people who had childhood asthma that apparently disappeared only to recur in later adulthood may have had quiescent asthma throughout that time, with some persistent airway inflammation and therefore airway damage. Much less is known about the long-term outcome of asthma in adults than in children.

One study did follow 181 adults with asthma,[2] and found that the patients who were youngest at diagnosis or who had received preventive treatment soon after diagnosis had no or less severe asthma 25 years later. This suggests that using long-term preventive treatment, even in mild asthma, improves its outcome. Neither the sex of the patient nor the presence of atopy appeared to be relevant prognostic predictors.

3.6 What happens to asthmatics whose asthma is well controlled?

One of the best predictors of future asthma control is past and present asthma control. The better asthma is controlled, the easier it is to maintain that control. The logical conclusion is that the persistent inhibition of airway inflammation leads to reduced airway hyperreactivity and less airway remodelling.

3.7 What happens to asthmatics whose asthma is poorly controlled?

Similarly, poorly controlled asthma implies poorly controlled airway inflammation and increased risk of long-term lung damage. Poorly controlled asthma has a worse prognosis and is more likely to result in airway remodelling and inevitable acceleration of the loss of lung function with age, and to an increased risk of the airway obstruction eventually becoming irreversible.

EFFECTS OF ASTHMA

3.8 What effect does having asthma have on patients?

Asthma is a very variable disease and ranges in severity from being nothing more than an occasional nuisance to being a severe life-threatening and life-dominating illness. It is relatively easy to determine the mortality from asthma and some of the more obvious examples of morbidity, but it is harder to measure the subtle effects of asthma that may alter the quality of many asthmatics' lives. Asthma is still associated with unacceptably high mortality and morbidity rates for such a common, well researched disease – for which there are such good, effective and safe treatments.

> One of the major aims of managing asthma is to abolish symptoms and to allow asthmatics to lead a normal life, minimally troubled by the disease or its management. For the majority of asthmatics, this ideal is achievable. Good asthma management should aim to give all asthmatics efficient and appropriate treatment so that they can become as near symptom-free as possible.

Large-scale representative surveys of asthma in the UK over the past few years have shown that there are still large numbers of asthmatics experiencing symptoms on a daily basis.[3,4] *See also Q. 2.4.*

The surveys have found that nearly half the respondents experienced symptoms on most days. Up to one-third of asthmatics were woken at least once a week by symptoms. Disturbed sleep in children may interfere with normal growth hormone secretion. A tired child may not fulfil its potential at school, and neither will a tired adult at work. This may have knock-on

TABLE 3.1 Effects of asthma			
Symptom	Short-term effects	Long-term effects	Implications
Reduced exercise ability	Reduced self-esteem	Failure to fulfil potential:	Loss to:
Wheeze or cough	Reduced self-confidence	• social	• individual
Night disturbance	Reduced physical fitness	• educational	• family
	Increased absenteeism	• economic	• community
	Reduced concentration	• occupational	• society
		• psychological	

effects for exams, promotion and self-esteem. Absenteeism from work due to asthma is a major problem, with nearly 25% of asthmatics taking up to one week off per year. This has social and economic consequences for the individual, the family and society as a whole. Amongst 9-year-old asthmatic children, one in eight loses more than 30 days from school because of the disease, again with potentially grave consequences for academic and developmental progress. Asthma symptoms can be very restrictive to leading a normal lifestyle. Most patients believe asthma restricts their daily lives, from avoiding smoky bars to choice of holiday locations, selection of employment (if possible), or even where to live.

The social costs of asthma are probably much higher. Some 25% of working asthmatics took more than one week off per year, with 8% stating they were unable to work at all due to asthma. A quarter of asthmatic children were reported as having more than two weeks off school due to asthma in the last year. One in three children and one in five adults were woken at least once a week by asthma.

Table 3.1 summarizes the effects of asthma symptoms.

Asthma also takes its emotional toll. Having any chronic disease may carry with it some emotional burdens: asthma is no different. The vast majority of asthmatics report that asthma has had some emotional impact on their lives. Many worry about the impact of asthma on their future lifestyle and well-being, and many expressed feelings of anger or guilt.

The more subtle effects on self-confidence and sense of well-being for asthmatics are impossible to calculate. The knock-on effects of this lack of confidence and poor self-esteem may result in underachievement and lack of fulfilment in education, personal relationships and employment.

3.9 What effect does having asthma have on the parents or carers and families of patients?

Children whose sleep is disturbed by coughing will wake themselves, and will almost certainly wake and worry their parents. Both child and parents run the risk of chronic tiredness and poor performance.

Adult asthmatics may wake themselves or their partners, again leading to chronic fatigue, irritability, poor concentration and impaired performance of both parties.

Poorly controlled asthma may lead to real or perceived disabilities by patients and their families. Lifestyle changes undertaken to reduce trigger exposure can have major implications for asthmatics and their families. Patients with more severe asthma or unstable asthma are a source of constant worry to their families.

3.10   How many people die from asthma each year?

Asthma is a major cause of premature death in the UK. In 1995, 1621 people were certified as having died from asthma;[5] in 1992, this figure was 1962. The numbers of deaths have been slowly declining since reaching a peak in the mid-1980s (*Fig. 3.1*). The age-standardized mortality rates from asthma in England and Wales fell by about 6% per year from 1983 to 1995 in people aged 5–64 years, with a slower decline in those aged 65 years and over. The

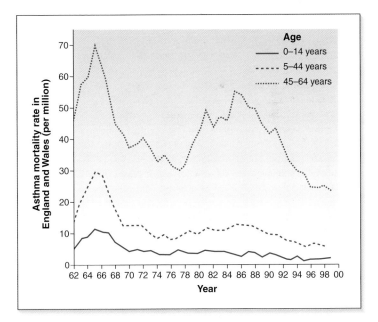

Fig. 3.1 Asthma mortality in England and Wales, 1962–2000. From National Asthma Campaign 2001,[9] with permission.

total number of deaths from asthma in people aged under 65 years fell by over 22% during this period.

Whilst these declines are encouraging, there is no room for complacency. Around 1500 people a year still die from asthma each year in the UK. The majority of these deaths are in the elderly, but 25 children and more than 500 adults aged under the age of 65 years died from asthma in the UK in 1999. Asthma therefore causes a disproportional loss of potential life, estimated as 35 000 years in 1991.

The recent decline in mortality from asthma might be due to the increased use of inhaled corticosteroids; a study from Canada clearly showed that asthmatics who took more than 400 micrograms of beclometasone daily were protected from death.[6] As inhaled steroids are used increasingly, it is hoped that there will be further reductions in the mortality rate for asthma. It is important to keep examining the trends in mortality, to report deaths, and to remember that asthma can still be a fatal disease. The mortality rate is continuing to increase in Japan and the USA, but has declined from peaks in the mid-1980s (as in England and Wales) in Australia, Germany and New Zealand.

Putting the number of asthma deaths in context, the approximate mortality rates of some diseases in the UK in 1999 were:

Ischaemic heart disease	150 000
Stroke	70 000
Breast cancer	12 000
Road traffic accident	4 500
Asthma	1 500

The accuracy in death certification for asthma has been under scrutiny. In one health district[7] 18 deaths were certified as being due to asthma, but on closer inspection seven of the 18 were clearly due to other causes and in one it was impossible to differentiate the exact cause of death. Indeed, applying stringent criteria to reporting of deaths due to asthma, it has been estimated that the true annual number of deaths due to asthma nationally is nearer 500.[8] Both in the UK and in the USA, death rates are much more likely in the poor than the rich. In England and Wales, there is a tendency for the mortality rate to rise with increasing distance from hospital.

3.11 Which patients are most at risk of fatal asthma?

Confidential enquiries suggest that many asthma deaths might have been prevented with adequate routine and emergency care. Factors associated with deaths from asthma in the UK include:

- Poor adherence to medication regimens
- Lack of ongoing medical care and lack of clear plans for recognizing and managing deterioration

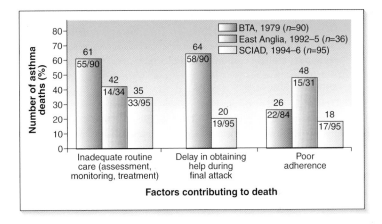

▲

Fig. 3.2 Some avoidable factors associated with death from asthma. BTA, British Thoracic Association; SCIAD, Scottish Confidential Inquiry Into Asthma Deaths. From National Asthma Campaign 2001,[9] with permission.

- ■ Poor patient education
- ■ Poverty
- ■ Patients whose first language is not English
- ■ Patients with poor social and emotional support
- ■ Patients with psychological factors including depression (*see Q. 1.18*).

The relative importance of some of these factors is detailed in *Fig. 3.2*.

COSTS AND CONSEQUENCES OF ASTHMA

3.12 What are the costs of asthma to the nation?

In 1997, the cost of asthma to the National Health Service (NHS) in the UK has been estimated at over £850 million a year. This is equivalent of about £500 per asthmatic. The bulk of this was on prescriptions for asthma medication, although there is some evidence that the increased prescription of preventive drugs helped to reduce the overall cost of treatment by contributing to effective asthma management and thus fewer acute asthma attacks. The cost of general practitioner consultations was estimated to be about £40 million a year.

The economic costs of asthma extend far beyond the price of the drugs used to manage the disorder. Indeed, the components of total cost can be classed under four main categories: direct medical resources, non-medical resources, indirect costs and psychosocial factors.

DIRECT MEDICAL RESOURCES

This is the cost of medical and nursing time used in diagnosing, treating and monitoring the illness. Included in the medical costs are all drug therapies, hospital outpatient appointments, accident and emergency attendances, hospitalization and other healthcare provider contacts.

NON-MEDICAL RESOURCES

These are costs directly associated with the illness but not relating to treatment by doctors or nurses. Examples include the costs of social support including home help, travel costs, waiting times and modifications to homes.

INDIRECT COSTS

These are the costs that result from the effects of asthma on the patient and the patient's family. They include the cost of absence from work or school (including parental time off to care for sick children), loss of productivity whilst at work or the complete loss of productivity resulting from death. In the UK, for example, some 17 million days were lost to asthma from work in 1994–5. This accounted for nearly 3% of all certified days lost in that period. The direct cost to the UK Department of Social Security in sickness and other benefits due to asthma was over £100 million, and the estimated loss of productivity has been put at over £500 million.

PSYCHOSOCIAL FACTORS

These are the costs for the patient or the patient's family, including the loss of work or other opportunities for the patient, loss of ability to engage in athletic pursuits, failure to fulfil educational, social or occupational potential, and a general diminution in quality of life. The social costs of asthma are much more difficult to quantify. Asthmatic patients are more likely to be unemployed than non-asthmatics, and most asthmatics believe that asthma limits their occupation. Some 50% of asthmatics say they have difficulty gaining promotion or have been previously dismissed from their job because of asthma. In addition, asthmatics in the UK have to face prescription charges, which can place a near intolerable burden on those who are just above the threshold for entitlement to free prescriptions. There may also be the cost of travel to and from hospital, as well as loaded life insurance premiums. No less important are the effects of the costs to the individual and society of lost potential. Social and other ambitions may have been unnecessarily limited, and personal fulfilment and happiness handicapped.

In 1997, the annual costs of asthma in the UK were calculated as £1226 million for lost productivity (55% of the total costs), £850 million for NHS costs (38%) and £161 million for social security costs (7%) – a total of £2237 million.[9]

The medical costs of asthma relative to total healthcare expenditure are actually quite small, accounting for less than 1% of the total UK health expenditure. The medical costs of asthma are less per capita than the cost of diabetes, heart disease or depression. On average, the medical care costs of asthma account for only about 50% of the total disease costs. The disproportion of this medical care is for emergency or rescue care.

In particular the non-medical costs are affected by the severity of asthma, being much less in mild to moderate disease but progressively more substantial as the disease increases in severity. The economic costs of asthma therefore extend well beyond the costs of therapy used to manage the illness. Indeed, it has been shown that patients randomized to inhaled steroids and β-agonists experienced significant improvement in lung function and symptom frequency compared with patients randomized to β-agonists and placebo or inhaled anticholinergic therapy.

The implications of such studies are that the increased costs of treating asthma with preventive drugs (normally inhaled corticosteroids) and the subsequent reduction in acute asthma attacks should be seen as an investment rather than as purely increased expenditure. The investment repays not only the patients in terms of quality of life, but also the nation in terms of reduced secondary costs and fulfilment of the national population's potential and less drainage on that nation's gross domestic product. The National Asthma and Respiratory Centre in the UK has estimated that one bed-day in hospital costs about £360 – more than the cost of inhaled high-dose steroids for one patient for a whole year.[10]

3.13 Does asthma get worse with age?

Factors associated with poorer prognosis of adult asthma are:

- Severe asthma
- Irreversible component
- Onset over the age of 40 years
- Negative skin test result
- Continuous exposure to occupational agents.

It has been established that the natural rate of decline in lung function with age is accelerated by asthma. Early treatment of asthma with inhaled steroids soon after diagnosis preserves lung function and, if applied to those with more severe disease, the inevitable rate of decline in lung function can be slowed by the addition of inhaled steroids (*see* Q. 3.5).[11]

It seems logical that delaying the institution of anti-inflammatory treatment may result in irreversible airway damage (*see Q. 3.4*).

3.14 Does smoking or occupation affect the prognosis of asthma?

After the age of about 25 years, lung function declines with age. This decline is accelerated in patients who smoke and who are susceptible to the adverse effects of smoking, and in patients with severe or poorly controlled asthma. Patients with severe asthma who also smoke risk an accelerated decline in lung function from both factors. Smoking also reduces the body's immune efficiency and smokers are at greater risk of respiratory infections and of developing chronic obstructive pulmonary disease. All of these factors mean that asthmatics that smoke are at greater risk of poorly controlled asthma, of accelerated decline in lung function and of developing irreversible airway obstruction.

Continued or repeated exposure to allergens and triggers may also worsen the prognosis of patients with asthma. Those with definite occupational asthma should be strongly encouraged to change their occupation or at least to minimize any future exposure to suspected or proven triggers (*see Q. 2.42*).

3.15 Can asthma cause long-term lung damage?

- Poorly controlled asthma accelerates the decline of lung function associated with ageing.
- Asthma can also cause airway remodelling and chronic scarring.
- The combination of these factors can lead to permanent lung damage.
- Good asthma control, using regular inhaled steroids, seems to mitigate against the long-term lung damage associated with poorly controlled asthma.

3.16 Do adults lose their asthmatic tendency?

Although asthma in adults is probably incurable, there are undoubtedly a significant number of asthmatics whose symptoms and signs of airway inflammation and obstruction have abated for many years. However, such patients may still show signs of airway hyperreactivity on bronchial challenge. Thus, although these patients may have lost their symptoms and signs, they have not completely lost their asthmatic tendency. Their symptoms may return at any time in the future; such patients should be alerted to this likelihood (*see Q. 3.5*).

3.17 What factors may lead to long-term improvements or deterioration of asthma?

In adults and children, one of the most exciting prospects in treating asthma is the possibility of reducing the long-term lung damage that may occur in badly treated or undertreated asthma by using early and full-dose preventive or protective therapy. Poorly treated or severe reversible obstructive airway disease (asthma) may eventually lead to long-term lung damage. The long-term use of inhaled steroids may help this trend. In children, vigorous treatment of infants at risk of developing asthma with inhaled steroids at their first presentation will reduce the sensitization and inhibit the subsequent severity of asthma.[2,10,11] *See also Q. 2.34*

Treatment and management of asthma

4

AIMS OF ASTHMA MANAGEMENT

4.1	What should I be aiming to do when managing patients with asthma?	86
4.2	Can we always meet these aims?	86
4.3	But isn't asthma a disease of exacerbations and remissions? Why can't I just treat the exacerbations?	86
4.4	How can I tell whether a patient's asthma is under good control?	86

TRIGGER AVOIDANCE AND ALLERGY THERAPY

4.5	Which triggers should a patient with asthma avoid?	87
4.6	What about skin prick tests – how useful are they?	87
4.7	What about desensitization – why don't we use this form of treatment in the UK?	88
4.8	But surely allergen avoidance must be important?	88
4.9	What advice can we give about animal avoidance?	89
4.10	Should all pets be banned from households where there is an asthmatic person?	89
4.11	Which families should be advised not to get new pets?	89
4.12	What about house dust mites?	90
4.13	What should we advise about trigger avoidance at work?	91
4.14	What about smoking and asthma?	91
4.15	What advice should we give about exercise?	91
4.16	Many patients say that pollution makes their asthma worse. How should we advise them?	91
4.17	Can changing diets help asthma?	92
4.18	What should asthmatics do about colds?	92

NON-PHARMACOLOGICAL TREATMENTS

4.19	Breathing, yoga and so on – are they of any use?	92
4.20	Should asthmatics be vaccinated against influenza every year?	93
4.21	Should asthmatics be offered pneumococcal vaccine?	93
4.22	Does physiotherapy have a role in the management of asthma?	94

MANAGING FACTORS ASSOCIATED WITH ASTHMA

4.23	Do ear or nose problems affect asthma control?	94
4.24	Does gastro-oesophageal reflux disease (GORD) affect asthma control?	94

PHARMACOLOGICAL TREATMENTS

4.25	What types of drug are available to manage asthma?	94

β_2-AGONISTS

4.26	How do short-acting β_2-agonists work?	95
4.27	How should we use them?	95
4.28	How often should we use them?	96
4.29	What are the side-effects of short-acting β_2-agonists?	96
4.30	What are the costs of short-acting β_2-agonists?	97
4.31	What are the differences between the different preparations?	97
4.32	Why not use short-acting β_2-agonists as the only treatment?	97
4.33	When should other agents be added in?	98

PREVENTIVE THERAPIES

4.34	What preventive agents are there?	98
4.35	Which agent should I choose first and why?	98

INHALED STEROIDS

4.36	Should all patients be on inhaled steroids?	99
4.37	At what age should young children and babies start on inhaled steroids?	99
4.38	What dose of inhaled steroids should I start with?	100
4.39	What dose of inhaled steroids is best for maintenance?	101
4.40	How do inhaled steroids work?	101
4.41	How well do inhaled steroids work?	101
4.42	What are the long-term benefits of inhaled steroids?	102
4.43	So when should inhaled steroids be started?	102
4.44	Do inhaled steroids show a dose–response?	103
4.45	What are the local side-effects of inhaled steroids?	103
4.46	What are the systemic side-effects of inhaled steroids?	104
4.47	What about children's growth and inhaled steroids?	106

4.48   Does the dose of inhaled steroid make any difference to children's growth?   106

4.49   What about the intermittent use of inhaled steroids for children – surely that makes sense?   107

4.50   Is there any difference between the different types of inhaled steroids?   107

4.51   Are inhaled steroids safe?   107

4.52   What are the overall benefits of early intervention with inhaled steroids in childhood asthma?   108

4.53   Can steroids cause asthma to remit?   108

4.54   Do inhaled steroids improve airway remodelling in patients with asthma?   108

ADDITIONAL TREATMENTS: OPTIONS

4.55   What treatment should I consider for patients whose asthma is not adequately controlled with regular use of inhaled steroids?   109

4.56   Which option is best?   109

4.57   What is the evidence in favour of adding long-acting β_2-agonists rather than increasing the dose of inhaled steroids?   109

LONG-ACTING β_2-AGONISTS

4.58   What long-acting β_2-agonists are available and what are their advantages?   110

4.59   Are there any disadvantages of long-acting β_2 agonists?   110

4.60   How are long-acting β_2-agonists used in practice?   111

4.61   When should high-dose inhaled steroids be used with inhaled long-acting β_2-agonists?   111

4.62   Are the effects of long-acting β_2-agonists plus inhaled steroids greater than the sum of the two components?   112

ORAL LONG-ACTING β_2-AGONISTS

4.63   What are oral long-acting β_2-agonists?   112

LEUKOTRIENE RECEPTOR ANTAGONISTS

4.64   How do leukotriene receptor antagonists (LTRAs) work?   112

4.65   How should LTRAs be used?   113

4.66   What are the advantages and disadvantages of using LTRAs?   113

THEOPHYLLINES

4.67	How do theophyllines work?	114
4.68	How should I use theophyllines?	114
4.69	What about the side-effects of theophyllines?	115
4.70	What blood level should I aim for?	115
4.71	What other factors affect blood levels of theophyllines?	115
4.72	Are there any other important drug interactions?	116

CROMOGENS

4.73	What are the cromogens and how do they work?	116
4.74	How should I use the cromogens?	117

ANTICHOLINERGIC AGENTS

4.75	How do anticholinergic agents work?	117
4.76	How are anticholinergic agents used in asthma?	118
4.77	Are anticholinergics of any use in infants and small children with asthma?	118
4.78	What about in the elderly?	118
4.79	Which patients should have which third-line therapies?	118

OTHER DRUG THERAPIES

4.80	What is the place of oxygen in the management of chronic asthma?	119
4.81	When should I use antibiotics?	119
4.82	What about using antihistamines for asthma?	119

ORAL STEROIDS

4.83	Which patients should have long-term oral steroids?	120
4.84	Are any precautions advised for people on long-term oral steroids?	120
4.85	When should the dose of oral steroids be tapered off?	121
4.86	How should the dose of oral steroids be tapered?	121
4.87	Should we prescribe long-term oral corticosteroids in primary care?	121
4.88	Are there any alternatives to long-term oral steroids?	122
4.89	What about vaccinations for patients taking oral steroids?	122
4.90	What about chickenpox in patients on oral steroids?	122

WHICH THERAPY?

4.91	What is the best therapy?	122
4.92	What regimens are there to manage asthma?	123
4.93	What is the step approach?	123
4.94	Where do I start?	124
4.95	So what are the BTS/SIGN steps?	124
4.96	What do I do if a patient has a short-term increase in symptoms?	127
4.97	Do I have to go up and down the steps one at a time?	127
4.98	When should a patient come back down from a temporary high step?	127
4.99	What do I do if the patient doesn't respond?	128
4.100	When should I step up long-term therapy?	128
4.101	When should I step down long-term therapy?	128
4.102	Why should I step down?	129
4.103	Does it matter if I step down too slowly or too quickly?	129

SELF-MANAGEMENT PLANS

4.104	What is a self-management plan?	130
4.105	Do self-management plans really help?	132
4.106	How can patients recognize deterioration?	133
4.107	Should all patients measure their peak flow every day?	133
4.108	How can patients know what to do if they think their asthma is getting worse?	133
4.109	What should patients do if they think their asthma is deteriorating?	134
4.110	So what peak flow levels are important?	134
4.111	When should patients call for help?	134
4.112	Which patients should have access to home oral steroids?	134
4.113	What type of steroid tablets should they have?	135
4.114	When should patients start their home steroids?	135
4.115	Should self-management plans be symptom or peak flow led?	135
4.116	Are there any examples I can use?	136

ACUTE ASTHMA

4.117	How can I recognize acute severe asthma?	136
4.118	What about acute asthma – which drugs do I use first?	137

4.119	If the patient responds, what do I do next?	138
4.120	What if the patient doesn't respond – what do I do then?	139
4.121	What about follow-up after an episode of acute asthma – when should I see the patient and what should I do?	139

INHALER DEVICES

| 4.122 | What types of inhaler device are there? | 140 |
| 4.123 | How do I decide which inhaler device to recommend? | 140 |

METERED-DOSE INHALERS

4.124	What are the advantages and disadvantages of metered-dose inhalers?	141
4.125	How do you use a MDI?	142
4.126	Should I replace all my patients' CFC-driven inhalers with HFA-driven ones?	142
4.127	Are there any differences in CFC- and HFA-driven inhalers? Which do patients prefer?	143

SPACERS

4.128	What about spacers – what types are there?	143
4.129	What are the advantages and disadvantages of spacers?	144
4.130	Which spacer should I recommend?	145
4.131	How should patients use spacers?	146
4.132	Do patients need to care for their spacers?	146
4.133	What about spacers in children with asthma?	146

BREATH-ACTUATED DEVICES

4.134	What are breath-actuated devices?	147
4.135	How do patients use breath-actuated aerosols?	147
4.136	What are the advantages and disadvantages of breath-actuated aerosols?	148

DRY POWDERED DEVICES

4.137	What are dry powdered devices?	149
4.138	How do patients use the dry powdered devices?	150
4.139	What are the advantages and disadvantages of dry powdered devices?	151

NEBULIZERS

4.140	How do nebulizers work?	153
4.141	What are the advantages and disadvantages of using nebulizers?	154
4.142	When should the routine use of nebulizers be recommended?	154
4.143	How should we deal with patients who already have home nebulizers?	155

CHOOSING A DEVICE

4.144	Which devices should we use for children?	155
4.145	Which devices should we choose for adults?	155
4.146	Which devices should we use for the elderly or disabled?	156
4.147	What about relative costs of asthma therapies?	157

PQ PATIENT QUESTIONS

4.148	Why should I need to take inhaled steroids for my asthma – surely it would be better to avoid whatever causes my asthma?	158
4.149	I find it very difficult to find the time and money I should be spending in trying to reduce the dust and mite exposure in my house. What should I do to help my daughter who has asthma?	158
4.150	How can I tell if my asthma is getting better or worse?	158
4.151	Are inhaled steroids safe even in children or if used over a long time?	159
4.152	Does it matter if I miss the occasional dose of my regular inhalers?	159
4.153	If steroids are so safe, why are sportsmen and women not allowed to use them?	159
4.154	How does my doctor or nurse know which treatment is right for me?	159
4.155	Will treating my asthma help make the disease go away, or will I need to take treatment all my life?	160
4.156	Will I get addicted to any of my treatments?	160

AIMS OF ASTHMA MANAGEMENT

4.1 What should I be aiming to do when managing patients with asthma?

The aims of asthma management are to:

- Recognize asthma
- Abolish symptoms
- Restore normal or the best possible long-term airway function
- Minimize the risk of severe attack
- Enable normal growth in children
- Minimize absence from school or work.

Children should expect to grow and develop normally, taking part in all the activities enjoyed by every other child. *See Q. 5.6 and Q. 5.7.*

4.2 Can we always meet these aims?

It may not always be possible to achieve every goal for every asthmatic. Nevertheless, these aims should always be clearly agreed with the patient, with modifications as necessary for certain asthmatics.

4.3 But isn't asthma a disease of exacerbations and remissions? Why can't I just treat the exacerbations?

Treatment is aimed at preventing exacerbations and protecting the lungs. Acute exacerbations – especially if requiring hospital admission, an out-of-hours consultation or nebulization – can usually be regarded as a failure of chronic management.

Preventive treatment should be the minimum that controls and maintains lung function so that the patient is free from exacerbations; relieving treatment should be whatever is necessary to keep the asthmatic symptom-free and able to lead a normal life. *See Q. 4.32.*

4.4 How can I tell whether a patient's asthma is under good control?

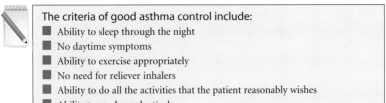

The criteria of good asthma control include:
- Ability to sleep through the night
- No daytime symptoms
- Ability to exercise appropriately
- No need for reliever inhalers
- Ability to do all the activities that the patient reasonably wishes
- Ability to work productively

- Peak flow readings stable and at best possible levels
- Ability to have a cold with impunity, and to tolerate exposure to common allergens and triggers including changes in the weather
- No exacerbations or fear of exacerbations – the patient can rely on stable control of the disease.

The mission statement of the Swindon Asthma Group is to try to ensure that: 'Every asthmatic should lead a normal life untroubled by their asthma or its management.'

TRIGGER AVOIDANCE AND ALLERGY THERAPY

4.5   Which triggers should a patient with asthma avoid?

Common triggers of asthma are ubiquitous and some are impossible to avoid. Initially it is important to listen to what an asthmatic may think are important triggers for them, and to discuss possible avoidance with the patient. It is important to stress that total avoidance and control is nearly impossible and that it is often easier to treat the effects rather than radically altering one's lifestyle. The degree of shifts in lifestyle will vary with the severity of the symptoms and personality of the asthmatic. It is important that parents are not made to feel responsible for their child's asthma or guilty that they aren't undertaking some of the quite drastic changes that are sometimes advocated for trigger avoidance. Any changes they do make must be the result of full and frank discussions with the patient and (if appropriate) the family, rather than as a result of an emotional reaction. Skin prick tests and radioallergosorbent tests (RASTs) can help to confirm suspected allergens. *See also Q. 1.6.*

4.6   What about skin prick tests – how useful are they?

Skin prick tests can be useful in determining whether an individual is likely to be allergic to specific allergens. They are most useful before contemplating any major lifestyle changes. An example might be if parents were contemplating getting rid of a loved household pet in trying to improve their child's severe asthma. However, the skin prick test should be recommended only in specific instances. Knowing that a patient has had a positive reaction to skin prick test is not in itself necessarily very helpful. Knowing that one might be allergic to something one can do nothing about does not help control the asthma. Skin prick tests are useful only if taken with a careful history. It is more important for a patient to avoid an allergen that they know from experience can upset their asthma, even though their skin prick test may be negative, than to rely totally on the skin prick test results.

Skin prick tests to most common allergens are available commercially and are fairly easy to use; full instructions come with the kits. They are eminently usable by practice nurses or general practitioners (GPs). The test kits can be purchased by GPs (they are not available on prescription in the UK) and need to be kept in the fridge. The kits have a limited shelf-life of a few years. The full kit costs about £100 and can be ordered through most pharmaceutical wholesalers. The kits contain ranges of allergens, such as common pollens and moulds, food additives and animal allergens.

Skin prick test results must be taken in conjunction with a full allergic history. Up to 40% of the population will test positive to an allergen if you screen for enough of them (*see Q. 2.20 and Q. 2.24*).

4.7 What about desensitization – why don't we use this form of treatment in the UK?

Immunotherapy or desensitization was a popular therapy in the UK until the mid-1980s, when the resulting mortality rate was considered unacceptable. It is still widely used in North America and the rest of Europe. The long-term efficacy of most desensitizing agents for asthma is still doubtful. Desensitization can induce an anaphylactic reaction and so should be undertaken only when full resuscitation can be safely carried out and the patient can be monitored for 2 hours after treatment. Immunotherapy can reduce symptoms caused by house dust mite, cat dander, and various moulds and pollens, but there has been no study that shows a reduction in the amount of medication needed to reduce asthma symptoms in the long term. Immunotherapy is best reserved for young patients with severe rhinitis and/or mild asthma that is induced by a few selected seasonal or perennial allergens (e.g. house dust mite). Immunotherapy is less effective in symptom reduction for patients with more severe asthma.[1,2] There are no unique benefits from immunotherapy that are not achievable by other interventions. A meta-analysis of clinical trials of immunotherapy[3] showed only modest effects in improved objective assessments in asthma and confirmed that allergen immunotherapy is a safe and long-term effective treatment option only in highly selected patients with allergic asthma.

4.8 But surely allergen avoidance must be important?

Most advances in the treatment of asthma have concentrated on suppressing the effects of the disease rather than eliminating the cause. This is because it is much easier to treat the asthma with preventive or relieving drugs, which are increasingly sophisticated and relatively free from side-effects, especially if taken by inhalation. Eliminating the causes of asthma is difficult. Few asthmatics have only one or two known causes and, even if they are known, it is often impossible to eliminate exposure to them.

This aspect of asthma management remains controversial. Whilst it is widely accepted that allergies are important in provoking asthma, it is not clear whether knowing which specific allergens provoke asthma in an individual will actually help with that individual's asthma care. Many allergens are impossible to avoid or exposure can be reduced only by drastic alterations in lifestyle – not only for the patient but their families too.
See also Q. 1.9.

4.9   What advice can we give about animal avoidance?

Animal allergens are usually in their urine, saliva or dander. All pets should be completely banned from all bedrooms all the time. Animal dander persists for up to six months after the removal of the animal from the bedroom, so allowing the cat in to sleep on a child's bed every two or three months is inadvisable. Washing the cat weekly can reduce its allergic potential. This sometimes has the unfortunate side-effect of making the cat run away. Don't get confused and put the cat in the freezer (*see Q. 4.12*)! Caged birds and mammals may be hidden triggers at school, although the importance of such exposure is probably minor. The removal of any caged bird or animal from bedrooms and living rooms is advisable.

4.10   Should all pets be banned from households where there is an asthmatic person?

Almost certainly not. Although a number of patients, especially children, may be sensitive to their pet, removal of the offending animal may not necessarily make much difference to the patient's asthma, as the animal is unlikely to be the exclusive trigger. If the patient's asthma is proving difficult to control and the patient is unable to live a normal lifestyle or has frequent exacerbations, or there is a danger to the patient's life or long-term health, then consideration of removing the family pet is justified. Any trial of pet removal must be absolute and continue for at least six months.

Having a pet is part of normal childhood for many families, and the animals provide great pleasure to their owners and family. The positive effects of pet ownership should never be underestimated, and nor should the effects of potential emotional trauma from losing a pet.

4.11   Which families should be advised not to get new pets?

Patients with a strong family or personal history of atopy, especially if triggered by animal exposure, should be careful before considering pet ownership. Positive skin prick tests or RAST results may help make the decision more straightforward (*see Q. 2.20 and Q. 2.2.1*).

4.12 What about house dust mites?

The house dust mite is ubiquitous, especially in modern, centrally heated homes with insulation, double glazing and fitted carpets. Exposure can be reduced only with some difficulty (*see Q. 1.8*). The optimal conditions for house dust mite are ambient temperatures of 25–30°C with 75–80% relative humidity. The full recipe for reducing exposure is as follows:

■ Remove all toys, pillows and other soft furnishings made from animal fibres. This can often cause distress to small children if their favourite cuddly toy is removed permanently. A compromise is to place the toy in the freezer overnight once or twice a week.

■ Use as new a mattress as possible. Use new pillows and duvets. Feathers and goose down have not been implicated in housing higher concentrations of house dust mites. The bedding should be washed in hot water (over 55°C), or dry-cleaned.

■ Cover the bedding with dust-mite impermeable covers. The mattress should be vacuumed on both sides and then placed in the cover, which should be zippered up and left. Ideally, start with a new mattress. When choosing a mattress cover, choose a full cover that completely encases the mattress and zips shut. Top-fitting covers can actually increase the amount of house dust mite residues that can be emitted from the mattress. Choose breathable covers, which prevent the build-up of humidity beneath them. The covers need damp dusting occasionally. They are quite expensive: some of the best cost nearly £100. Although impractical for most people, the fitting of air-conditioning or living in a tightly built home with ventilation exhaust systems can also help drastically to reduce the house dust mite concentration.

■ Remove the carpet in the bedroom and use floorboards with rugs or cushion flooring, or ideally straw mats.

■ Ascaridal agents are no more effective than continuous house dust mite avoidance measures alone.

■ Undertake damp dusting, but take care not to increase the interior humidity too much; good intensive vacuuming, especially with filters, can also be helpful.

■ Ventilate the bedroom daily.

■ Wash the curtains every six months at high temperature (more than 55°C) or, better still, replace them with blinds. Keep the windows open as much as possible to air the house and keep the humidity low (under 60%), although this may increase the level of airborne allergens such as pollen.

If all the above measures are applied assiduously, the house dust mite concentration can be reduced by up to 10 000 times. However, it is unclear whether this results in consistent clinical benefit. Indeed, most children with asthma do not derive sufficient benefit for this type of treatment to be of relevance to them, bearing in mind that these treatments are time consuming, costly and extremely inconvenient. This finding was confirmed in a meta-analysis of 23 randomized controlled trials that had investigated the effects on asthma patients of chemical and physical measures to control house dust mites, or both. The conclusions from the pooled results of studies showed that current methods of trying to reduce exposure to these allergens are ineffective and cannot be recommended as prophylactic treatment for asthma patients sensitive to house dust mites.[4]

4.13 What should we advise about trigger avoidance at work?

Once a susceptible person has been sensitized, subsequent exposure to even very low levels of sensitizer can trigger asthma symptoms. A large number of substances have been implicated (*see Table 1.1*). It can often be impossible for a worker to continue in their employment without exposure to the trigger for their asthma. Whether to treat or change jobs needs to be discussed with each individual.

The management of occupational asthma is discussed more fully in *Q. 5.65*.

4.14 What about smoking and asthma?

Children born to mothers who smoke during pregnancy are more likely to have asthma, and antenatal smoking results in higher cord blood immunoglobulin E. The incidence of wheezing in children can be related to the amount of smoking by their mothers. Smoking is a common trigger for many asthmatics of all ages. For that reason, both parents should stop smoking before starting a family. No child should ever be exposed to any second-hand cigarette smoke, and certainly no asthmatic should ever smoke (*see Q. 1.16*).

4.15 What advice should we give about exercise?

For the majority of people, normal recreational exercise is enjoyable and beneficial to their health. Regular exercise should be encouraged for all asthmatics at all ages. It is usually best to use drug treatment to allow appropriate exercise, rather than reduce the need for drugs by forced inactivity and prohibiting what should be an essential part of life.

Exercise will improve overall physical fitness and well-being, but will not greatly improve lung function.

4.16 Many patients say that pollution makes their asthma worse. How should we advise them?

Exposure to smoke, sprays and polishes at home should be kept to a minimum. It is difficult for an individual to do much about air pollution.

Air pollution is usually perceived as a greater problem than it is, as discussed in *Q. 1.12 and* Q. *1.13*. Moving to a less polluted area is rarely an option. For patients with asthma sensitive to outdoor pollution, local environmental factors (including prevailing winds from other possibly polluting sites and future local plans for industry or commerce) should be considered when any house moves are contemplated. Masks, ionizers, humidifiers and dehumidifiers are of no proven benefit. Many patients do get symptomatic relief from cool, fanned air.

4.17 Can changing diets help asthma?

Dietary manipulation rarely modifies asthma. Occasionally an asthmatic will be sensitive to specific additives such as sulphite, a preservative used in beer, or to wine, dried fruit or processed potatoes. Reduced exposure of infants to allergens in food can reduce the frequency of allergic disorders in the first years of life. There have recently been some suggestions that a diet rich in oily fish leads to a lower prevalence of asthma than expected, and a high sodium intake has been linked to higher rates than expected. Fresh fruit consumption also appears to have a beneficial effect on lung function in children. In practice, it seems sensible to advocate a 'healthy', well-balanced diet that includes plenty of fresh fruit and vegetables without making claims for specific foods. (*See Q. 1.31.*)

4.18 What should asthmatics do about colds?

These are nearly always viral and are one of the most common triggers cited by asthmatics (*see Q. 1.7*). At the first sign of such an infection it is important to monitor the peak flow and symptoms. For some time now it has been considered orthodox to tell the patient to double the dose of their preventive therapy and to use their relievers more liberally, but there is little firm evidence to support this practice and it should now be abandoned. It is sensible for those with more severe or unstable asthma to try to avoid contact, if possible, with other people suffering from heavy colds, influenza or other viral illnesses.

NON-PHARMACOLOGICAL TREATMENTS

4.19 Breathing, yoga and so on – are they of any use?

Homeopathy, yoga, hypnosis, acupuncture and chiropractic all have their advocates. There have not been many good controlled trials of these complementary therapies, but certainly acupuncture, chiropractic and transcendental meditation have been shown to be ineffective. The Buteyko technique is a system of breathing exercises intended to improve asthma control. The theory is difficult to marry with conventional understanding of the physiology of respiration, and there have been no proper trials of this technique. The great danger of these therapies is that the proven and effective drug treatments may be stopped and the protective effect of preventive treatments will be lost, leading to chronic persistent subclinical airway inflammation and perhaps dangerous unstable asthma.

Yoga may help some people by teaching control of breathing and relaxation techniques, but it has no effect on airway inflammation or hyperreactivity and should be used as an adjunct to conventional therapy, not as a replacement.[5]

An analysis of 15 randomized controlled trials has shown that there is no evidence of efficacy from mental or muscular relaxation techniques, hypnosis, biofeedback techniques or autogenic training.[6]

Other non-drug therapies, such as air filters and ionizers, have been shown to make no difference in asthma. The use of non-feather pillows has actually been shown to be positively associated with childhood wheeze, even after adjusting for all other factors.

4.20 Should asthmatics be vaccinated against influenza every year?

Influenza vaccination is recommended every autumn for all patients with severe asthma, or for any asthmatic aged 60 years or more, or for patients who have asthma in addition to other illnesses such as chronic obstructive pulmonary disease, diabetes, heart disease or kidney disease. Influenza exacerbates respiratory problems and can cause considerable morbidity and mortality. The most recent UK epidemic was in 1989–90, when an estimated 29 000 deaths resulted. Modern influenza vaccines give at least 80% protection against influenza strains related to those in the vaccine. The vaccine is prepared each year from strains that the World Health Organization predicts will be most prevalent later in the year. There are few side-effects: local soreness and transient febrile myalgia or arthralgia are the commonest. The only contraindication is a history of anaphylactic reaction to previous vaccines or to eggs (although some brands of vaccine are not manufactured using egg proteins – check with the manufacturer before offering the vaccine to a patient with a clear history or documentation of anaphylactic reaction to eggs). Oral steroid treatment, even long term, is not a contraindication. Very few children will benefit from influenza vaccination.

4.21 Should asthmatics be offered pneumococcal vaccine?

Pneumococcal vaccine is also recommended for the same group of patients as influenza vaccination. *Streptococcus pneumoniae* is a major cause of pneumonia (especially in those at risk), bacteraemia and meningitis. Patients with more severe asthma or mixed obstructive airway disease are at particular risk of infection. Pneumococcal pneumonia affects about 1 in a 1000 adults annually, with a mortality rate of 10–20% of those infected. The vaccine is virtually without side-effects and the only contraindication is pregnancy. A single vaccination is said to offer lifelong immunity, unless the patient has had a splenectomy, in which case advice from a local specialist should be sought.

Influenza and pneumococcal vaccine can be given at the same time.

4.22 Does physiotherapy have a role in the management of asthma?

Physiotherapy may be a useful addition to pharmacotherapy and leads to improvements in exercise tolerance and quality of life. Many patients with asthma tend to hyperventilate, probably because they perceive a small change in airway resistance as being much greater than it is. Such patients may subconsciously breathe more rapidly and shallowly in response to a variety of stimuli. Control of breathing and diaphragmatic stretching exercises can help such patients.

MANAGING FACTORS ASSOCIATED WITH ASTHMA

4.23 Do ear or nose problems affect asthma control?

Undoubtedly. One of the commonest reasons for asthma that is difficult to control is severe or undertreated rhinitis. The irritability of the upper airway mucosa and increased nasopharyngeal mucus production leads to increased lower airway irritability, increased bronchial hyperreactivity, and worsening symptoms and control of asthma. Conversely, impeccable control of a patient's rhinitis usually helps in the control of a patient's asthma and may be a prerequisite for that control. There is a strong association between asthma and rhinitis, especially but not exclusively in atopic patients. Nasal polyps are often found in atopic seasonal or perennial rhinitis.

There are also associations between otitis media and asthma, and again good control of either condition will improve the control of the other.

4.24 Does gastro-oesophageal reflux disease (GORD) affect asthma control?

Yes, in some cases. There is an association between asthma and GORD, and poor control of either disorder may lead to worsening control of the other. Good control of GORD may be a prerequisite for good control of the asthma, and vice versa.

PHARMACOLOGICAL TREATMENTS

4.25 What types of drug are available to manage asthma?

Of all the common chronic conditions that are managed mainly in the community, none has the range, specificity, safety profile and quality of medications available for treatment as has asthma. The range of treatments available and different ways of using them are confusing to doctors, nurses and patients.

> **There are eight types of drugs used to treat asthma:**
> 1 β_2-agonists (short-acting)
> 2 Corticosteroids
> 3 Cromogens
> 4 β_2-agonists (long-acting)
> 5 Theophyllines
> 6 Anticholinergic drugs
> 7 Leukotriene receptor antagonists
> 8 Other drugs (*see Appendix A*).

The preferential route for asthma medication is by inhalation. This allows small amounts of active drug to be applied directly to the lining of the bronchus, so small doses of drugs can be used that work quickly with minimal systemic bioavailability.

β_2-AGONISTS

4.26 How do short-acting β_2-agonists work?

These drugs are bronchodilators that stimulate the β_2-adrenergic receptors in the bronchial smooth muscle, producing relaxation of the muscle. They also enhance mucociliary clearance and decrease vascular permeability. In general, their activity lasts for approximately 4 hours.

They can be given by inhalation using aerosols or dry-powdered devices, or nebulizer, or by tablets, syrup or injection.

4.27 How should we use them?

■ Short acting β_2-agonists are the treatment of choice for the relief of symptoms of asthma. They can also be used just before exercise to prevent exercise-induced asthma.

■ All asthmatics should have a short-acting β_2-agonist, preferably given by inhalation. Ideally, they should seldom be needed.

■ Short-acting β_2-agonists may be the only treatment needed for mild asthma. However, there is increasing evidence that there is an inflammatory element in even mild asthma. This means that preventive treatment should be the treatment of choice in all but the mildest cases. The frequency with which a short-acting β_2-agonist is used is a good marker of asthma control.

■ The regular, frequent use of β₂-agonists as the *only* treatment may mask the underlying decline in lung function that may occur in some asthmatics not treated with preventive agents.

4.28 How often should we use them?

Ideally, patients with stable well-controlled asthma will not need to use their short-acting β₂-agonist at all, or very seldom.

Short-acting β₂-agonists can be used every 4 hours or so in worsening or severe asthma. They are the treatment of choice for the relief of symptoms and reversal of bronchospasm. In acute, severe asthma they can be used every 3 hours or so.

They can also be taken to prevent exercise-induced asthma, when they should be used 10–30 minutes before the start of exercising.

A potential problem is that the misuse of short-acting β₂-agonists alone to provide a rapid bronchodilator response and control of frequent symptoms can result in the patient relying on their bronchodilator alone, when in fact they should also be using regular anti-inflammatory therapy. Reliance on the strong symptom-suppressing effects of the short-acting β₂-agonists might delay the use of necessary anti-inflammatory drugs, leading to accelerated airway remodelling and decline in lung function, and also to increased sensitivity of the airways, especially of the β₂-receptor sites. The net result is more unstable, more severe, asthma with a poorer prognosis.

4.29 What are the side-effects of short-acting β₂-agonists?

Inhaled drugs

These have very few side-effects. Some susceptible individuals may experience tremor (the commonest side-effect), headaches or tachycardia. The side-effects are dose related.

Oral drugs

Side-effects are usually mild and transient. Palpitations, tremor and tachycardia are the most common. Cramp and headaches may occur, as may low blood potassium levels. Use oral short-acting β₂-agonists with caution if the patient also has thyrotoxicosis, poorly controlled heart failure or cardiomyopathy. Occasionally small children may show behavioural disturbances, usually hyperactivity, when given oral bronchodilators. A very few children seem to react in this way, and may even experience such behavioural changes with short-acting inhaled β₂-agonists.

4.30 What are the costs of short-acting β_2-agonists?

Inhaled drugs are very cheap, especially when given by metered-dose inhaler. Other devices may be more expensive, but may provide more reliable delivery.

Oral preparations are very cheap.

4.31 What are the differences between the different preparations?

The inhaled route is to be preferred if at all possible. There is little to choose between the main inhaled preparations salbutamol (albuterol) and terbutaline; the choice of inhaler device is probably more important than the choice of preparation. Orciprenaline is a less selective β_2-agonist than the other two.

Oral preparations are used less frequently because they have greater risks of side-effects and a slower onset of action compared with inhaled preparations. There are no major differences between salbutamol (albuterol) and terbutaline syrups or tablets.

4.32 Why not use short-acting β_2-agonists as the only treatment?

Since the 1980s there have been fears that the regular use of the short-acting β_2-agonists would be associated with increased morbidity and mortality from asthma. There is a significant relationship between short-acting β_2-agonist over-use and death, especially when the β_2-agonist is administered by nebulization. This relationship probably reflects the severity of the underlying asthma and misuse of the drug rather than an inherent danger from the drug itself.

Epidemics of deaths from asthma occurred in the 1960s in many countries, including the UK, where a high-dose preparation of isoprenaline was readily available. Mortality fell after withdrawal of the over-the-counter preparation. A further epidemic occurred in New Zealand in the 1970s involving the drug fenoterol.

There is also evidence that the regular use of short-acting β_2-agonists leads to an increase in the rate of decline in lung function, but, although this was shown after two years,[7] the effect was less easy to demonstrate after four years.[7] Regular use of short-acting β_2-agonists also leads to increased variability in peak flow during treatment and slight increases in bronchial hyperreactivity after cessation of the treatment.

The effectiveness of short-acting β_2-agonists as bronchodilators is not disputed, but there still remains some concern that they may worsen asthma control if they are used regularly and that excessive use may increase the risk of death from asthma. Excessive short-acting β_2-agonist use by asthmatics definitely indicates an increased risk of severe asthma and suggests the need for anti-inflammatory medication.

4.33 When should other agents be added in?

■ The British Thoracic Society/Scottish Intercollegiate Guidelines Network (BTS/SIGN) guidelines[9] www.sign.ac.uk/guidelines recommend that patients who need to use short-acting β_2-agonists more than once a day for relief of symptoms require the administration of other agents, preferably regularly inhaled steroids.

■ Many other authorities and guidelines would recommend the use of regularly inhaled steroids if short-acting β_2-agonists were being used more than two or three times a week.

■ Any patient who has had a recent exacerbation (an increase in symptoms over several days requiring repeated doses of inhaled short-acting β_2-agonists, especially if they also needed oral steroids or nebulized therapy, or if the patient attended an emergency department or was admitted to hospital) should be considered for additional preventive therapy. The more severe or frequent the exacerbation, the stronger the case for starting additional preventive therapy.

■ If the short-acting β_2-agonists are being used only for the prevention or relief of exercise-induced asthma, and they are not needed for symptom relief otherwise, it is perfectly acceptable to allow more frequent use of these drugs as the only treatment for asthma. All other patients should receive regular preventive therapy.

PREVENTIVE THERAPIES

4.34 What preventive agents are there?

■ Inhaled steroids
■ Inhaled cromogens (cromoglicate or nedocromil)
■ Leukotriene receptor antagonists (oral).

4.35 Which agent should I choose first and why?

Inhaled steroids should be the first choice. They are recommended by all major guidelines including those of the BTS/SIGN[9] (www.sign.ac.uk/guidelines) and the Global Initiatives for Asthma (GINA).[10] The evidence for their efficacy in symptom and disease control is very strong. Inhaled steroids are very safe as well as very effective for long-term use. They are by far the most effective form of preventive therapy available for the management of asthma.

For the minority of patients who are unable or unwillingly to comply with regularly inhaled steroid therapy, *inhaled cromogens* can be tried. However, they are not as effective as inhaled steroids, need to be taken more frequently, and take longer to reach the peak of their effectiveness.

Patients who fail to respond or whose asthma is still imperfectly controlled after 4–6 weeks of therapy with regularly inhaled cromogens should switch to regularly inhaled steroids.

The third group of drugs available for first-line asthma control or prevention are the *leukotriene receptor antagonists* (LTRAs). LTRAs are licensed and used in this way in the USA, but in the UK are currently licensed only as add-on therapy for patients already using inhaled steroids or cromogens, or for patients with 'pure' exercise-induced asthma. Although very effective in some patients, LTRAs are less so in others, and the concern remains that they may not show the disease-modifying attributes of the inhaled steroids.

INHALED STEROIDS

4.36   Should all patients be on inhaled steroids?

Many clinicians would advocate this view, arguing that asthma is a chronic, incurable, inflammatory disease that requires chronic anti-inflammatory therapy for adequate control in the long term.

This view is logical and difficult to dispute; however, there are two groups of patients for whom regular, long-term use of steroids may not be indicated. These patients are also extremely unlikely actually to use twice-daily treatment in the long term, in the absence of symptoms or disability:

■ The first group includes those with 'pure' exercise-induced asthma. There is no evidence of airway inflammation in this group of patients and so long-term inhaled steroid use is not indicated.

■ The second, larger, group comprises those patients with very mild asthma whose symptoms are very intermittent and whose lifestyles are hardly compromised by their having asthma. Even though we clinicians may tell these patients that they have a chronic inflammatory lung condition that may decline more quickly without regular use of inhaled steroids, and that there are perhaps potential dangers from unopposed chronic airway inflammation, the patients are unlikely to adhere to any treatment that requires them to take regular treatment for a condition that rarely troubles them and for which the threat of future difficulties is distant and unproven.

4.37   At what age should young children and babies start on inhaled steroids?

Although there is good evidence that the earlier inhaled steroids are started the better, in terms of preventing long-term airway damage and irreversible loss of lung function there is little evidence to guide us in deciding at what age to start inhaled steroids.

From the point of view of their beneficial effects, inhaled steroids should be started at as young an age as possible. From the point of view of possible problems with inhaled steroids being used in young babies, the clinician needs to consider the possible effects on lung maturation and lung growth, as well as other potential side-effects as detailed in *Q. 4.45 and Q. 4.46*.

As a practical compromise, it seems sensible to start long-term inhaled steroids in babies with a probable diagnosis of asthma from the age of 1 year; below this age, referral to a consultant paediatrician, preferably with an interest in asthma, is advised. The younger the child, the stronger the advice to seek a second opinion.

4.38 What dose of inhaled steroids should I start with?

Surprisingly, there is no consensus on the optimum starting dose of inhaled steroids. Historically, the advice was to start with the lowest possible dose and gradually to increase it until optimum control was reached. This advice reflected the suspicions about inhaled steroid safety prevalent when they were first introduced. The main problem with this approach was that it often took many weeks to bring about good control of a patient's asthma. In the interim, the patient was still suffering, and was also at risk of losing faith in the treatment being advocated.

Subsequently, many clinicians advised starting on a high dose of inhaled steroids, trying to achieve good control of the asthma as quickly as possible (and keep the patient's faith) and then slowly reducing the dose to the minimum that controlled the patient's asthma. The main problem with this approach is that many patients are not adequately monitored once control has been achieved and are left on higher doses of steroids than they may need – often indefinitely.

The current approach reflects aspects of both former approaches. Start at the dose appropriate to the severity of the patient's asthma. The starting dose should be in the middle to lower range for the patient's age and severity of symptoms or airflow limitation. This reflects our current understanding of the dose–response to inhaled steroids as well as the importance of adhering to regular, effective inhalations of steroids at the most cost-effective doses.

As a guide:

- *Adults*: beclometasone or budesonide 200–800 micrograms (μg)/day; flunisolide 500–2000 μg/day; fluticasone 100–400 μg/day; mometasone 200–400 μg/day; triamcinolone 200–800 μg/day.
- *Children*: beclometasone or budesonide 100–400 μg/day; flunisolide 500–1000 μg/day; fluticasone 50–200 μg/day; mometasone 50–200 μg/day; triamcinolone 100–400 μg/day.

4.39 What dose of inhaled steroids is best for maintenance?

The maintenance dose will usually be the same as the starting dose. There is no need to increase the dose of inhaled steroids in most patients, and there is little point in doing so as the dose–response curve of these drugs usually reaches a maximum at 200–800 µg/day beclometasone, or equivalent. The patient should be monitored and the criteria of good control applied, and additional therapy added as needed if control is still inadequate. (*See Q. 4.95.*)

4.40 How do inhaled steroids work?

Steroids suppress inflammation in asthmatic airways, although the precise molecular mechanism is not yet certain. They act on the cell nucleus and inhibit, in particular, the production of cytokines, thereby reducing the chronic inflammation in asthmatic airways. Steroids bind to specific receptors in the cells of the airway epithelium and in the endothelium of bronchial vessels. From the receptor, the steroid moves to the nuclear compartment of the cell, where it exerts its main effects. The full effects on improving the functional abnormalities in asthma may take up to two weeks, and the full anti-inflammatory effects up to eight weeks. Inhaled steroids control the underlying inflammation and thereby reduce the severity and frequency of acute attacks, and reduce hyperresponsiveness of the bronchial airways, so leading to better day-to-day control of asthma.

4.41 How well do inhaled steroids work?

Studies have shown that after three months of therapy with inhaled steroids there is a reduction in the number of inflammatory cells seen in bronchial biopsy specimens.[11] Inhaled steroids have also been shown to reduce airway responsiveness. Prolonged treatment with inhaled steroids is effective against exercise-induced asthma.

Inhaled steroids significantly enhance the rate of increase in lung function in asthmatic children compared with that in asthmatic children not receiving inhaled steroids. This effect on lung function is greater when the steroid is started earlier after the asthma was diagnosed, so that children started early on inhaled steroids have significantly better lung function than those where steroid use is delayed until some years after the onset of asthma symptoms. Regular long-term use of inhaled steroids in children not only improves functional status and decreases sleep disturbance, but is also associated with a decreased burden on the parents.[12]

In summary, inhaled steroids should be used as first-line therapy in the treatment of even mild asthma, and inhaled steroid therapy should be initiated soon after diagnosis and continued long term. This allows not only good control of the asthma whilst the therapy is being taken but holds out the promise of modification of the disease process and a better prognosis in the future. The long-term use of inhaled corticosteroids may prevent the long-term damage to the lungs that might otherwise occur. Inhaled steroids are the drugs of choice for good control of most patients with asthma.

4.42 What are the long-term benefits of inhaled steroids?

■ Long-term treatment with inhaled steroids reduces airway responsiveness in asthmatic adults and children. The reduction in responsiveness takes place over several weeks and may not be maximal for three months or even longer.

■ For inhaled steroids to suppress inflammation in the long term, they need to be used regularly to maintain their control of the condition. If inhaled steroids are discontinued after only a few weeks of treatment, the airway responsiveness and symptoms soon return to pretreatment values.

■ Prolonged use of inhaled steroids can lead to complete resolution of airway inflammation, especially if the steroid therapy is started early in the course of the disease. Inhaled steroid therapy may therefore 'switch off' the disease process and lead to a complete resolution of asthma, even if the steroid therapy is later withdrawn.

■ Further evidence for the disease modification effect of inhaled steroids has been shown in studies that provided evidence that the rate of decline of lung function is slowed by the long-term use of inhaled steroids in both adults[13] and children.[14]

■ More recent research has shown that inhaled steroids improve airway remodelling in chronic asthma, but that the use of inhaled steroids needs to be prolonged (for several years at least).[15]
See also Q. 2.34.

4.43 So when should inhaled steroids be started?

There have been many studies showing the benefit of using inhaled steroids as soon as the diagnosis of asthma has been made or is being contemplated:

■ A Canadian study[16] showed that regular, prolonged use of inhaled steroids can result in marked improvements in symptoms and bronchial hyperreactivity in patients with what would usually be considered to be mild, controlled asthma. These improvements were accompanied by significant improvements in clinical status.

■ A Dutch multicentre study[17] showed that delayed intervention with inhaled therapy is less effective than immediate intervention.

■ A Finnish study[18] compared the effects of inhaled steroid therapy with those of a short-acting β_2-agonist alone in adult patients with newly diagnosed asthma. In its second phase, the study compared the effects of changes in therapy after the first two years of treatment.

The results of these studies showed that first-line treatment with an inhaled corticosteroid for two years resulted in a long-term improvement in asthma, which subsequently could be maintained for at least a year by a smaller dose of steroid – and in some patients even by placebo. The patients who were first treated with a short-acting β_2-agonist for two years and only subsequently with an inhaled steroid reached, on average, only half the level of lung function in the third year as those treated with an inhaled steroid from the beginning of the study. The authors concluded that some functional reversibility may be lost by delaying the start of steroid treatment. This is consistent with the known failure of short-acting β_2-agonist drugs to affect the underlying airway inflammation in asthma when used alone.

A Canadian study[19] has further confirmed the advantages of early steroid intervention. The authors concluded that regular treatment with inhaled steroids following the diagnosis of asthma can reduce the risk of admission to hospital for asthma by up to 80%.

4.44 Do inhaled steroids show a dose–response?

One of the most important facts to remember when prescribing inhaled steroids is that the maximum dose–response for most patients is reached at doses of 200–800 µg/day beclometasone, or equivalent.

Remember that the risk of systemic steroid activity is dose-dependent, so increasing the dose of an inhaled steroid will increase the risks of side-effects (admittedly still a small risk) and the costs of the medication, while not necessarily increasing the therapeutic effects.

4.45 What are the local side-effects of inhaled steroids?

Local side-effects are not necessarily dose-dependent, but are usually related to poor inhaler technique or to the type of inhaler.

The commonest unwanted effects of inhaled steroids are effects caused by the deposition of inhaled steroid on the mouth and pharynx. These effects include hoarseness of the voice, candidiasis (thrush) of the mouth or throat, and sore throat, throat irritation or coughing.

■ *Hoarseness* of the voice may occur in up to a third of patients receiving inhaled steroids; the incidence is related to the total dose of inhaled steroid rather than the dose frequency. Symptoms subside when inhaled steroids are withdrawn but may recur when treatment is reintroduced. Unlike most of the other local side-effects of inhaled steroids, the use of large-volume spacers does not appear to protect against dysphonia.

■ *Oral candidiasis* or thrush is seldom a major problem clinically. The incidence of positive throat swabs for *Candida albicans*, however, is much higher and can be well over 50%. Oral thrush seems to be much less of a problem in children. Oral thrush is more likely with higher-dose inhaled steroids and when the inhaled steroid is used four times daily instead of twice daily. Large-volume spacers appear to protect against oral thrush, but mouth rinsing does not seem to be beneficial.

■ *Cough and throat irritation* are common symptoms associated with the use of inhaled steroids, but the symptoms are less frequent if a dry-powder device is used.

4.46   What are the systemic side-effects of inhaled steroids?

The systemic side-effects of inhaled steroids are dose related.

> At the usual therapeutic doses of 200–800 µg/day beclometasone or equivalent, there are rarely any clinically important systemic side-effects from long-term use of inhaled steroids.

The benefits of inhaled steroids in asthma are very clear. However, even after 30 years of clinical use, there are still concerns about the systemic effects of inhaled steroids, especially as they are likely to be administered over long periods. It must be emphasized that, despite extensive studies over the past 30 years, the number of clinically important systemic side-effects – even from high-dose inhaled steroids – are very, very few. All studies need to evaluate the clinical relevance of detectable systemic effects rather than measurable changes in biochemical values, which may or may not be relevant. The systemic effect of an inhaled steroid will depend on the dose delivered to the patient, the extent to which the drug is metabolized in the liver, and inherent differences in responses between different patients.

EFFECTS ON ADRENAL FUNCTION

Treatment with steroids may suppress the production of adrenocorticotrophic hormone (ACTH), which in turn leads to reduced cortical secretion by the adrenal gland. This sequence of events will occur only if a significant amount of inhaled steroid is absorbed systemically. The vast majority of studies have failed to detect any adverse effects with doses of inhaled steroids of less than 1000 µg/day beclometasone, or equivalent, in adults on cortical secretion. Similarly, daily 1500 µg doses of inhaled steroids have not shown any deleterious affect on the hypothalamic–pituitary–adrenal axis.

The use of very high-dose inhaled steroids (far exceeding the manufacturers' maximum recommended doses) has been associated with an unexpected increase in acute adrenal crises, especially in children taking very high-dose fluticasone. Patients, especially children, should not be prescribed inhaled steroids in excess of those recommended by the manufacturers (1000 µg/day in adults, 400 µg/day in children for fluticasone). No case of clinical adrenal insufficiency has ever been reported in patients treated with inhaled steroids given at the recommended doses.

EFFECTS ON BONE METABOLISM

At present there are no indications that long-term treatment with inhaled corticosteroids is associated with increased rates of osteoporosis or fracture in children or adults. However, inhaled steroids can induce changes in laboratory indices of bone turnover in adults, although it is unclear to what extent such changes signify a clinically important risk of fracture after long-term usage of inhaled steroids. The position is further complicated by the fact that bone densitometry may be less sensitive and reliable in steroid-induced osteoporosis in predicting the risk of fracture compared with involutional osteoporosis. In children the suppression of biochemical indices of bone formation and resorption that is seen with oral prednisolone has not been seen with inhaled steroids.

EFFECTS ON THE SKIN

Oral and topically applied steroids may affect the skin, producing thinning, easy bruising, striae and telangiectasia. Skin thickness has been shown to be much reduced in patients receiving oral steroids compared with controls; those receiving long-term high-dose inhaled steroids have a skin thickness between the two groups. The presence of purpura was also shown to be commonest in those on oral steroids, less common in those on high-dose inhaled steroids, and least common in those not on any form of steroid. Patients receiving inhaled steroids report easy bruising more frequently than those who are not taking inhaled steroids. There are no reports of adverse effects of inhaled steroids on the skin in children.

EFFECTS ON THE EYES

Many studies have shown that inhaled steroids do not increase the risk of cataracts in children. In adults there is a weak link between the risk and severity of cataracts and the dose of inhaled steroids. There is an association between atopy and the development of cataracts, irrespective of any treatment for the manifestations of the atopy.

OTHER EFFECTS

There have been a few isolated case reports of behavioural and psychological changes in patients receiving inhaled corticosteroids. These changes occurred within the first two days and the symptoms improved on discontinuation of the drug. A few patients were able to tolerate lower doses of the same drug. Inhaled steroids do not suppress cellular immunity.

There is little evidence that inhaled steroids have any clinically relevant metabolic effects in either adults or children at the doses commonly prescribed.

4.47 What about children's growth and inhaled steroids?

The effects of inhaled steroids on growth are difficult to evaluate, partly because children with moderate or severe asthma seem to have a different growth pattern to that of normal children. These children tend to grow more slowly in early adolescence but they may continue to grow for longer than children without asthma, so that the final height of mature adults aged 20 years or more is roughly similar to that of of their peers. Those children with the most severe asthma may not ever achieve a normal height, irrespective of whether they have received corticosteroids at all. The height of asthmatic children not receiving steroids correlates significantly with the pulmonary function of these children, suggesting that asthma severity affects growth more than the treatment of that severe asthma.

There have been many controlled longitudinal studies with carefully selected control groups of asthmatic children that are used to assess the influence of inhaled steroids on growth. All these studies have concluded that the treatment of asthmatic children with inhaled steroids for up to five years with doses of as great as 800 µg per day does not adversely affect growth. No longitudinal growth studies have demonstrated any significant growth retardation in children treated with inhaled steroids.

Children with asthma will ultimately reach normal height and weight.[20] Those who are mildly affected tend to be even taller and heavier than adolescents without asthma. The severity of the asthma is a more important influence on final growth. Indeed, the addition of inhaled steroids when treating asthmatic boys may improve their growth rate. A large case–control study found that the attained heights of adults whose childhood asthma had been treated with inhaled steroids were no different from the attained heights of adults not so treated.[21]

4.48 Does the dose of inhaled steroid make any difference to children's growth?

Controlled studies involving more than 700 children have concluded that treatment with inhaled steroids for up to five years at doses as great as

800 µg per day does not adversely affect growth. Children's growth is therefore not affected by long-term use of inhaled steroids, irrespective of the dose, up to 800 µg a day of budesonide or equivalent.

4.49 What about the intermittent use of inhaled steroids for children – surely that makes sense?

There is some evidence that temporary, short-term, growth suppression occurs in children within the first few weeks of starting inhaled steroids. Over several weeks, growth will 'catch up', so that there is no long-term effect on growth. Using intermittent courses of inhaled steroids therefore confers no advantages on an asthmatic child, but has distinct disadvantages of leaving the child's airways exposed to the risk of unopposed inflammation (and potential long-term remodelling and permanent damage) and of causing recurrent dips in growth, which may carry a risk of long-term growth suppression.

4.50 Is there any difference between the different types of inhaled steroids?

In the UK, the available inhaled steroids are beclometasone, budesonide, fluticasone and mometasone. In other countries, including the USA, triamcinolone and flunisolide are also available for the treatment of asthma. There have been few studies comparing the efficacy of different steroids in the same patients, and none comparing the long-term effects of different inhaled steroids. However, the differences between the types is not likely to be of major significance, and there is little to choose between the available choices in terms of side-effects and efficacy, although fluticasone is about twice as effective as the same dose of budesonide and beclometasone.

4.51 Are inhaled steroids safe?

In summary, the side-effects of inhaled steroids are few and far between. I would emphasize the lack of evidence over the past 30 years of clinically significant side-effects for this very effective form of treatment. Indeed, the controversies over the use of inhaled steroids resolve around the issue of whether clinical benefit (which is abundantly clear) is justified in the face of the possible risk of long-term systemic complications such as osteoporosis, cataracts, adrenal suppression and growth inhibition. However, current evidence firmly suggests that the risk of such toxicity is not likely to be associated with the long-term use of at least 800 µg/day beclometasone, or equivalent, in adults or 400 µg/day in children.

4.52 What are the overall benefits of early intervention with inhaled steroids in childhood asthma?

Early intervention with inhaled steroid therapy in childhood asthma may have many benefits:

■ Reducing the risks of undertreatment and hospitalization.
■ Better long-term clinical control.
■ Allowing a lower life-time cumulative steroid dose than later intervention.
■ Probably reducing the risk of development of irreversible airway obstruction.
■ Not associated with any clinically important side-effects if used wisely.

4.53 Can steroids cause asthma to remit?

In many patients whose asthma is controlled with steroids there is a deterioration in asthma control within months of stopping the steroid treatment,[22] but some have not relapsed even when followed for up for one year.[23] Therefore, it seems that inhaled steroids suppress the underlying mechanism of asthma, producing remission of the condition in many of the patients so treated.

Better results are achieved, however, in studies on patients with mild to moderate asthma treated early and for a long time with inhaled steroids. This holds out the promise that prompt treatment with inhaled steroids soon after diagnosis, and continuation of such treatment over a relatively long time, may result in a better outlook for that individual's asthma.

There is good evidence[24] that asthma alone is quite capable of inducing irreversible airflow obstruction by causing structural changes in the walls of the airways, or airway remodelling. These changes may occur early in the course of the disease. Structural changes in the airways are seen even in patients with very mild, occasional symptoms, suggesting that airway remodelling is likely to affect all asthmatics, not just those with severe disease. The structural changes in the airways probably occur more slowly or are prevented altogether by the regular use of inhaled steroids, which should be started as soon as possible after diagnosis, even in 'very mild' asthma. *See also Q. 2.34 and Q. 4.42.*

4.54 Do inhaled steroids improve airway remodelling in patients with asthma?

Almost certainly, but the inhaled steroid therapy needs to be prolonged (for years) to be effective.

ADDITIONAL TREATMENTS: OPTIONS

4.55   What treatment should I consider for patients whose asthma is not adequately controlled with regular use of inhaled steroids?

Before making any changes in any treatment, it is essential to check the patient's inhaler technique and compliance. If control is still poor, consider adding:

■ Inhaled long-acting β_2-agonists.

If control is still inadequate, consider regular use of:

■ Additional oral leukotriene receptor antagonists (LTRAs)
■ Additional oral theophyllines
■ High-dose, inhaled, short-acting β_2-agonists
■ Higher-dose steroids. Try high-dose inhaled steroids first; if unsuccessful, consider oral steroids – but only after referral to a hospital specialist.

4.56   Which option is best?

There is now a wealth of evidence that adding inhaled long-acting β_2-agonists to regularly inhaled steroids is far more effective than higher doses of the inhaled steroids. The combination of regular use of inhaled steroids plus long-acting β_2-agonists is the optimal treatment for many asthmatics whose asthma is imperfectly controlled with inhaled steroids alone.

4.57   What is the evidence in favour of adding long-acting β_2-agonists rather than increasing the dose of inhaled steroids?

■ The original paper by Greening et al[25] showed that adding salmeterol to beclometasone (200 µg twice daily) significantly improved symptoms and peak flow readings compared with findings in patients randomized to higher-dose inhaled steroids.
■ Woolcock and co-workers[26] conducted a similar study, but the subjects had inadequately controlled asthma despite receiving 500 µg beclometasone twice daily at the start of the trial. The addition of salmeterol produced a more rapid and more pronounced beneficial effect on symptoms and lung function than doubling the dose of inhaled steroids.
■ Adding long-acting β_2-agonists to regular inhaled steroids produces superior improvements than adding LTRAs or theophylline.
■ The Formoterol And Corticosteroid Establishing Therapy (FACET) study[27] showed that adding formoterol (eformoterol) to either low- or high-dose inhaled steroids produced improvement in symptoms and lung function, but also reduced exacerbation rates by up to 61%.

Exacerbations fell from an initial average of 0.9 exacerbations per patient per year in the conventional-dose steroid group, to 0.34 per patient per year in the group treated with formoterol and high-dose steroids.

■ A meta-analysis of trials comparing the addition of salmeterol with increased dosage of inhaled steroids showed reduced exacerbation rates;[28] this benefit is not found if short-acting β_2-agonists are substituted for the long-acting β_2-agonists.

LONG-ACTING β_2-AGONISTS

4.58 What long-acting β_2-agonists are available and what are their advantages?

This class of drug includes long-acting inhaled bronchodilators such as salmeterol xinafoate or formoterol fumarate.

SALMETEROL

This agent is a bronchodilator whose duration of action is independent of the concentration used. Salmeterol has a long lipophilic side-chain that binds non-competitively to a part of the β_2-receptor. This means that salmeterol persists at the site of action for a sustained period, which accounts for its duration of action being longer than that of, for instance, salbutamol (albuterol). Salmeterol provides protection against bronchoconstriction that is long lasting and significantly greater than the protection provided by drugs such as salbutamol (albuterol). In children, salmeterol also produces effective bronchodilatation for up to 12 hours, and protects against exercise bronchoconstriction.

FORMOTEROL (EFORMOTEROL)

Formoterol (named eformoterol in the UK) is a competitive β_2-agonist whose long duration of action is dependent on the concentration used and its high affinity for the β-receptor sites in the airways. In the FACET study of patients who had persistent asthma symptoms despite regular inhaled steroids, the addition of formoterol improved lung function and symptoms, as did increasing the dosage of inhaled steroids. However, there was a significant fall in the rates of severe and mild exacerbations (26% and 40% respectively) when formoterol was added to conventional-dose inhaled steroids, and a further, dramatic, fall in the exacerbation rates (63% and 62% respectively) in patients treated with formoterol and high-dose inhaled steroids.[27]

4.59 Are there any disadvantages of long-acting β_2 agonists?

They are relatively free of side-effects and have low potential toxicity compared with long-acting oral β_2-agonists or theophyllines.

> Tremor, palpitations and headache may occur rarely.

There is no evidence of the bronchodilator effect declining with prolonged regular use.

4.60 How are long-acting β_2-agonists used in practice?

- These drugs are used when symptom control is still poor despite the adequate use of inhaled steroids, or as an alternative to increasing the dose of inhaled steroids in those still having symptoms despite receiving low doses of inhaled steroids. They are also used when night-time symptoms are particularly prominent but the control of the asthma is otherwise satisfactory.
- They are also useful for protection against exercise-induced asthma. In such cases they can be taken in the morning to protect against symptoms brought on, for instance, by a child with a gymnastics class in the morning and football after school.
- Long-acting inhaled β_2-agonists are given for their protective effect against bronchospasm and should not be used for immediate relief of acute symptoms, for which short-acting inhaled β_2-agonists are required. Similarly they should not be used as the sole protective treatment, but always in combination with inhaled corticosteroids or other regular anti-inflammatory agents. However, the introduction of long-acting inhaled β_2-agonists may not only improve lung function and symptom control, but also allow a reduction in the inhaled steroid dosage needed to maintain such improvements.
- Salmeterol is useful for adults and children aged four years and over. Formoterol (eformoterol in the UK) is useful in adults and children aged six years and over.

4.61 When should high-dose inhaled steroids be used with inhaled long-acting β_2-agonists?

High-dose inhaled steroids should be reserved for patients whose asthma is proving difficult to control despite good compliance and inhaler technique, and who are using or have tried all other therapeutic options – the option of high-dose inhaled corticosteroids may delay or prevent the need for long-term oral steroids. The dose of inhaled steroids should be increased to beclometasone 400–1600 µg twice daily, or equivalent, and if necessary fluticasone up to a maximum of 1000 µg twice daily. Referral to a specialist should be considered, especially in children; this recommendation is stronger in younger children and babies. High-dose inhaled steroids may also be used in patients already on long-term oral steroids if they permit a reduction in the dosage of the long-term oral steroids.

4.62 Are the effects of long-acting β₂-agonists plus inhaled steroids greater than the sum of the two components?

The evidence is overwhelming that the addition of long-acting β_2-agonists to inhaled steroids results in improved asthma symptoms without loss of asthma control. There is therefore an apparent additive interaction between the two compounds. As well as relaxing smooth muscle cells in the airways, long-acting β_2-agonists may also have some anti-inflammatory actions, mainly by potentiating the effects of inhaled steroids. The full therapeutic benefit of long-acting β_2-agonists requires the concomitant presence of inhaled steroids, as this counteracts the β_2-receptor desensitization that may otherwise occur if long-acting β_2-agonists are used alone. Recent experience has shown that using a product that combines an inhaled steroid with a long-acting β_2-agonist has greater therapeutic benefit than when the two components are used consecutively. The explanation is that the distribution of both products at a cellular level will be the same for the combination product, whereas when the products are given separately their cellular distribution will not exactly match.

ORAL LONG-ACTING β₂-AGONISTS

4.63 What are oral long-acting β₂-agonists?

Long-acting oral β_2-agonists are also available as slow-release salbutamol or terbutaline tablets, or as intrinsically long-acting bambuterol tablets.

> Long-acting oral β_2-agonists are far more likely to be associated with side-effects (tremor, palpitations, tachycardia) than the inhaled preparations.

There is no evidence that the oral preparations have the increased efficacy of the inhaled long-acting β_2-agonists. The use of oral long-acting β_2-agonists is confined to the few patients who cannot or will not take any form of inhaled therapy.

LEUKOTRIENE RECEPTOR ANTAGONISTS

4.64 How do leukotriene receptor antagonists (LTRAs) work?

These drugs have both anti-inflammatory actions (independent of and additional to those of corticosteroids) and bronchodilating actions (independent of and additional to those of β-agonists). Leukotriene antagonists inhibit the bronchoconstrictor effect of leukotrienes that is associated with allergens, exercise and cold air. The onset of their anti-inflammatory action resulting in clinical improvements in a patient's asthma is quicker than for inhaled steroids – 24 hours as opposed to several days – so they may be a more logical choice as intermittent therapy to cover, for example, exacerbations or likely exacerbations due to upper respiratory tract infection or temporary changes in an asthmatic's environment.

4.65 How should LTRAs be used?

LTRAs appear to have a good effect in mild to moderate asthma, with a reduction in nocturnal symptoms and in asthma exacerbations. They may also have a place in more severe asthma that is not adequately controlled with inhaled steroids. Neither high-dose inhaled steroids nor oral steroids are able to inhibit the increased leukotriene production in asthma. However, it is still not clear whether anti-leukotrienes are able to suppress the inflammatory response in asthmatic airways in the same way as inhaled steroids can, or whether they simply relieve symptoms by pure bronchodilatation, like the β_2-agonists. Their bronchodilating effect is as great in patients not using inhaled steroids as it is in those using long-term inhaled steroids. Montelukast and zafirlukast are licensed in the UK for the prophylaxis and treatment of chronic asthma, and in the USA as first-line maintenance therapies.

The response to LTRAs is very heterogeneous: a few patients show dramatic improvements using these drugs, but many appear to derive little or no benefit.

4.66 What are the advantages and disadvantages of using LTRAs?

One of the main advantages of leukotriene therapies is that they can be given orally. Montelukast can be given to adults and children over the age of 4 years; zafirlukast can be given to adults and children over the age of 12 years.

Side-effects of LTRAs

Side-effects are very few. Zafirlukast may infrequently cause changes in liver enzymes that require monitoring. Otherwise, the LTRAs appear to be well tolerated, with headaches and sore throats being the commonest side-effects. Tolerance and rebound worsening of asthma do not appear to occur. There are possible interactions between warfarin, aspirin, erythromycin and aminophylline with zafirlukast.

LTRAs are useful in atopic asthma, especially if the patient also has troublesome rhinitis, where the drugs may benefit the control of both the asthma and the rhinitis.

They are particularly helpful in controlling asthma in patients who are aspirin sensitive.

There is a slight concern that the use of LTRAs is associated with Churg–Strauss syndrome. This is a rare form of allergic granulomatosis that affects mainly young men and is characterized by peripheral nerve lesions, abdominal pains, skin rashes, ulcers or nodules, upper respiratory tract inflammation, eosinophilia, anaemia, high erythrocyte sedimentation rate and diarrhoea. There has been a slight increase in the incidence of the syndrome in patients taking LTRAs, but the association is probably not specific for LTRAs and may be a reflection that these patients had such a syndrome anyway but it was being suppressed by the high-dose steroids needed for asthma control. Adding a LRTA to their drug regimen allowed a reduction in the steroid dose and failure to continue suppressing the Churg–Strauss syndrome.

THEOPHYLLINES

4.67 How do theophyllines work?

The precise mechanism of their action is unclear. Theophyllines have some bronchodilator actions and some central stimulant actions, and also some anti-inflammatory actions. The latter effect may depend on the ability of the drug to regulate the influx and activity of inflammatory cells into the airways. These anti-inflammatory actions probably occur at doses lower than those commonly prescribed. Theophyllines probably have an immunomodulatory action as well, also at doses lower than those commonly prescribed.

4.68 How should I use theophyllines?

Theophyllines have a narrow therapeutic range. If the dose is too high and the resulting blood level also becomes too high, a variety of potentially serious side-effects may occur. Despite this, theophyllines may be useful for night symptom suppression, especially if given as a long-acting formulation, although they are less effective than salmeterol in preventing nocturnal asthma symptoms. They are much more widely used in North America than in the UK, where they are usually regarded as third- or fourth-line agents.

Theophyllines can be given parenterally to terminate acute severe asthma, preferably under electrocardiographic control. They can also be given orally, as medicines or capsules, or rectally. They are usually given as a liquid formulation or capsules. The main disadvantage is that they cannot be given by inhalation.

They are fairly cheap, although the sustained-release preparations are a little more expensive. Although theophyllines are cheaper than inhaled long-acting β_2-agonists, they are not as effective in the long-term control of asthma. The cost of measuring blood levels and of monitoring interactions, as well as the cost of poorly controlled asthma, may actually mean that theophyllines are not a cheaper alternative in the long run.

Sustained-release preparations are better for the relief of nocturnal symptoms. The dose often needs to be titrated against the effect, with regular monitoring of blood levels. The bioavailability of theophylline from different preparations is not equivalent, so do not swap brands unnecessarily. Theophyllines are best prescribed by their brand names, for this reason.

4.69   What about the side-effects of theophyllines?

- Side-effects are relatively common and include nausea, vomiting, tachycardia, arrhythmias, insomnia, seizures and sudden death.
- The effects are all much less common at therapeutic doses, so regular monitoring of blood levels is recommended.

- More recently there has been interest in using theophyllines at technically subtherapeutic doses, and continuing them if there is a good clinical response.
- Rapid-release preparations have a high risk of side-effects associated with rapid absorption.
- Intravenous administration should not be attempted unless the patient is connected to a cardiac monitor and full resuscitation facilities are available, because the risk of cardiac arrhythmia is considerable.

4.70   What blood level should I aim for?

For satisfactory bronchodilatation, a plasma theophylline concentration of 20 mg/L is required. Concentrations below 10 mg/L may be effective in some patients; empirical trials in individual patients are the only way of finding out.

Adverse effects occur more frequently and more severely at concentrations over 20 mg/L.

4.71   What other factors affect blood levels of theophyllines?

Blood levels can be affected by:

- Other illnesses, especially heart failure and liver disease
- Pregnancy

■ Other drugs, as detailed below
■ Smoking and nicotine replacement preparations
■ Diet.

The half-life of theophyllines is increased by the following, leading to higher plasma concentrations:

■ Heart failure
■ Cirrhosis
■ Viral infections
■ Old age
■ Drugs – allopurinol, antifungals (fluconazole, ketoconazole), calcium channel blockers (diltiazem, verapamil and possibly others), cimetidine, ciprofloxacin, clarithromycin, erythromycin, fluvoxamine and oral contraceptives.

The half-life of theophyllines is decreased by the following, leading to lower plasma concentrations:

■ Smoking and nicotine replacement products
■ Chronic alcoholism
■ Drugs – barbiturates, carbamazepine, phenytoin and rifampicin, St John's wort.

4.72 Are there any other important drug interactions?

There is an increased risk of hypokalaemia with concomitant use of oral corticosteroids, diuretics and oral β_2-agonists, and a much smaller risk with regular high-dose β_2-agonists especially in the presence of hypoxia. The risks of hypokalaemia are thus greatest in acute asthma.

CROMOGENS

4.73 What are the cromogens and how do they work?

These drugs comprise disodium cromoglicate and nedocromil sodium. They are preventive agents that have weak anti-inflammatory actions, mainly at a cellular level. They act by inhibiting the release of chemical mediators from inflammatory cells, especially mast cells. Nedocromil may produce some reduction in airway responsiveness.

Cromogens have no bronchodilator action. Cromoglicate has no effect against any allergic response that is already in progress, unlike corticosteroids which do have such an action. Nedocromil is no more effective or better tolerated than cromoglycate or inhaled steroids, and therefore has no role in first-line management of mild to moderate asthma.

Cromogens should be used only as preventive therapies. They have some prophylactic action against exercised-induced symptoms. Nedocromil may provide some protection against virus-induced exacerbations of asthma.

They are not as effective in controlling asthma symptoms as inhaled steroids, and there is no evidence that they offer any long-term advantages at all when compared with the undoubted long-term benefits of inhaled steroids.

Generally, inhaled steroids are preferable to cromogens. The only use of cromogens is for patients who refuse to take regularly inhaled steroids.

4.74 How should I use the cromogens?

Cromoglicate may be useful in children, especially those with allergic type asthma. It is less useful in adults. It is difficult to predict accurately which children will most benefit. A 6-week trial is required to determine efficacy. *Nedocromil* can be used only in children over the age of 6 years.

Either drug may be useful when inhaled steroids cannot, or will not, be used by patients despite good education. However, their general anti-inflammatory properties are weaker than those of inhaled steroids, and for that reason the inhaled steroids remain the anti-inflammatory drug of choice for the vast majority of asthmatics. Apart from being less effective than inhaled steroids, the other main disadvantage of cromoglicate and nedocromil is that they must be taken at least three or four times daily to be effective. This clearly creates problems with compliance and with needing to use them at work or school.

A randomized placebo-controlled study in children aged 4 years or under showed that cromoglicate was no more effective than placebo.[29]

ANTICHOLINERGIC AGENTS

4.75 How do anticholinergic agents work?

These agents are bronchodilators that block the postganglionic vagal pathways, so reducing vagally induced bronchoconstriction. They tend to be less effective in asthma than β_2-agonists and act more slowly. They can be used by inhalation only.

> Side-effects are rare except at high doses. Anticholinergic agents should be used with caution in patients with glaucoma. Some patients do not like the taste, and some get a dry mouth when using them.

Anticholinergics are fairly cheap. Ipratropium is shorter acting than oxitropium, which is more expensive.

4.76 How are anticholinergic agents used in asthma?

With the exceptions listed below, these drugs have little or no part to play in the routine management of most patients with asthma. They are used as an alternative to β_2-agonists in the few patients who are very sensitive to the side-effects of β_2-agonists.

Often anticholinergic agents are used in patients who have chronic obstructive pulmonary disease (COPD) with a reversible component, or 'mixed asthma–COPD', as many patients with COPD find anticholinergic therapy alone or combined with short-acting β_2-agonists more effective than β_2-agonists alone.

They may have an additive effect when nebulized together with β_2-agonists in acute asthma.

4.77 Are anticholinergics of any use in infants and small children with asthma?

Although they are traditionally used in the routine management of infants and babies with asthma, there is no good evidence that anticholinergics are superior or safer than β_2-agonists.

4.78 What about in the elderly?

Anticholinergic therapy is no more effective or safer than β_2-agonist therapy in the elderly, but many patients with COPD find anticholinergic therapy more effective, and others find that a combination of the two works best. Elderly patients with asthma derive no additional benefit from anticholinergics but, given the difficulties in accurately distinguishing 'pure' asthma from mixed asthma–COPD, many elderly patients are given combination bronchodilator therapy or just anticholinergics. In practice, therapeutic trials of each therapy given individually and in combination can be tried for each patient.

4.79 Which patients should have which third-line therapies?

All patients who are still symptomatic, or who need frequent administration of short-acting β_2-agonists (more than once a day), or whose peak flows are still suboptimal or unstable despite good compliance and inhaler technique, and who are using regular inhaled steroids and long-acting β_2-agonists should be given a third-line therapy.

Third-line therapies include theophyllines, anticholinergics, LTRAs and oral steroids.

OTHER DRUG THERAPIES

4.80   What is the place of oxygen in the management of chronic asthma?

Although long-term oxygen therapy is of undoubted value in the management of severe COPD with respiratory failure, few patients with asthma will benefit from home oxygen treatment.

Many asthmatics derive some symptomatic benefit from oxygen, but there is a large placebo effect. The cooling effect from the flow of oxygen can also be soothing, but may be achieved more safely, cheaply and easily by using an electric fan. Allowing a few patients with very severe asthma access to occasional use of cylinder oxygen may give them some symptomatic relief but can also be quite expensive, and should never be a substitute for proper asthma management.

Long-term home oxygen therapy should never be prescribed in primary care unless the patient has been fully investigated, including arterial blood gas measurements, and has had a properly conducted trial of oxygen.

Chronic respiratory failure is rare in asthma. If it is suspected (chronic central cyanosis, palmar erythema, flapping tremor, dilated peripheral veins), refer to a respiratory specialist.

4.81   When should I use antibiotics?

Antibiotics are often given in acute exacerbations of asthma. They have a very limited role but may help to clear an associated sinusitis. Acute exacerbations of asthma may result in the production of green or yellow sputum, but this does not necessarily imply infection. Antibiotic treatment of associated infections such as sinusitis must not be seen as a treatment for asthma. Antibiotics should never be given in preference to specific asthma therapy in acute exacerbations. Antibiotics have no role to play in the routine management of asthma. They should be reserved for clinically apparent pneumonias or sinusitis, usually with local and systemic symptoms and signs including fever and dyspnoea. An increase in asthma symptoms accompanied by coughing up green or yellow sputum implies airway inflammation and not necessarily airway infection.

4.82   What about using antihistamines for asthma?

The use of antihistamines is an attractive proposition, especially in patients with allergic asthma. Histamine is one of the main chemical mediators in the allergic asthmatic process. However, it is only one of a number of mediators, and the use of antihistamines in acute asthma and chronic asthma has proved disappointing. The routine use of antihistamines in asthma is therefore not recommended.

ORAL STEROIDS

4.83 Which patients should have long-term oral steroids?

- Only those whose asthma control remains inadequate despite good compliance and inhaler technique, and who are already using maximum therapeutic doses of their current drugs.
- Patients should be using high-dose inhaled steroids plus inhaled long-acting β$_2$-agonists, and have had full therapeutic trials of LTRAs and theophyllines.

4.84 Are any precautions advised for people on long-term oral steroids?

Systemic steroids may have severe and important side-effects, which are usually dose-related as detailed in *Q. 4.46.*

SKIN

Long-term oral steroid treatment can result in thinning of the skin and increased bruising. Patients should be told to take care of their skin, using moisturizers and emollients as necessary.

METABOLIC

Oral steroids undoubtedly suppress the hypothalamic–pituitary–adrenal axis, and the degree of suppression is dependent on the dose of steroid given. This suppression may last for many months after oral steroid therapy has been stopped. Patients should be told never to stop their long-term oral steroid therapy suddenly, but always to do so under medical supervision.

BONE METABOLISM

Systemic steroids can induce osteoporosis by increasing bone absorption and decreasing bone formation. This osteoporosis is clinically important in that a large proportion of patients receiving long-term oral steroids will experience vertebral or rib fractures. All patients on long-term oral steroids need to discuss osteoporosis prevention and be offered bone densitometry scans at regular intervals. Liaison with local rheumatologists is advised.

4.85 When should the dose of oral steroids be tapered off?

 If oral steroids are used for 21 days or less, there is no need to taper off the dose. There is no evidence, even in children, of adrenal suppression if four or fewer courses of oral steroids are given per year, each of less than 21 days.

4.86 How should the dose of oral steroids be tapered?

Courses that are longer than outlined above, or if the course is repeated within six weeks of a previous one, or when trying to stop long-term oral steroids, require slow, gradual, tapering down of the dose. Tapering should be slower and more gradual if the oral steroids have been used for longer times.

Reductions may vary from a 5 mg reduction at daily intervals to a 5 mg reduction at weekly or fortnightly intervals.

If a patient has been on oral steroids for years, reduce very slowly (down to a 1 mg reduction every 2–4 weeks) and monitor peak flows and symptoms throughout the period of reduction and for 3–6 months afterwards.

4.87 Should we prescribe long-term oral corticosteroids in primary care?

There will undoubtedly be a few asthmatics who require regular long-term oral steroids – perhaps 1–2% of all asthmatics on a GP's list. Before deciding on this therapy, confirm that:

■ The diagnosis is correct
■ The patient is complying with all their asthma therapy and has good inhaler technique
■ All the other therapies are being used at their maximum therapeutic doses.

Unless you feel confident about managing asthma and monitoring patients on long-term oral steroids, referral to a chest physician when contemplating such a step is advisable.

Referral to a paediatrician with expertise in managing asthma is strongly advised before committing any child to such therapy.

4.88 Are there any alternatives to long-term oral steroids?

The folic acid antagonist methotrexate has been used in severe steroid-dependent asthma. Unfortunately its potentially serious side-effects (especially myelosuppression and mucositis) outweigh any beneficial effects in asthma. Similarly, the immunomodulators azathioprine and ciclosporin may produce some small clinical benefit in patients with the most severe asthma, but again there are very severe potential side-effects (myelosuppression and hepatotoxicity with azathioprine; nephrotoxicity with ciclosporin). Use of all these drugs should be initiated and monitored only by hospital specialists.

4.89 What about vaccinations for patients taking oral steroids?

This is a difficult problem, but only for live vaccines. Live vaccines are contraindicated in individuals who may be immunosuppressed, such as those taking high-dose oral steroids, because these individuals may suffer overwhelming infection as a result of the live vaccination. If at all possible, postpone live vaccination until at least three months after stopping the oral steroids. If the oral steroids cannot be stopped, refer to a specialist in infectious diseases or immunology for further advice.

Children taking long-term oral steroids should already be under the care of a paediatrician, and such questions should always be addressed to them.

The live vaccines commonly used in the UK are:

- Polio
- Rubella
- Measles (MMR)
- BCG (tuberculosis).

4.90 What about chickenpox in patients on oral steroids?

Fatal varicella (chickenpox) can occur in patients susceptible to it who are on oral steroids even in the short term. If such a patient is exposed, stop the steroid if possible and give zoster immunoglobulin and oral aciclovir if varicella develops. If infection with chickenpox is suspected, immediate hospital treatment is required.

WHICH THERAPY?

4.91 What is the best therapy?

Most patients will be well controlled on regular inhaled steroids with inhaled bronchodilators as needed. For the majority of patients not so controlled, additional regular use of long-acting β_2-agonists with regularly inhaled steroids provides exceptional control because both the inflammatory process and its consequences are continually inhibited. This combination is not only logical but is effective, and results in fewer exacerbations as well as better symptom control.

In summary:
- *Mild asthma* – regular use of inhaled steroids with inhaled short-acting β_2-agonists as needed.
- *Moderate asthma* – regularly inhaled steroids plus regular use of inhaled long-acting β_2-agonists, with inhaled short-acting β_2-agonists as needed.
- *Severe asthma* – regular use of inhaled steroids plus inhaled long-acting β_2-agonists plus oral theophyllines, with inhaled short-acting β_2-agonists as needed.

4.92 What regimens are there to manage asthma?

There are many published regimens for the management of asthma.[9,10,30]

Management is based on the patient's symptoms and peak flow readings (if possible). The severity of a patient's asthma is classified according to which therapies are needed to control the asthma. The regimens recommended by GINA and the BTS/SIGN (www.sign.ac.uk/guidelines) are similar; the latter are described in more detail here as an example of the stepwise approach to successful asthma management.

4.93 What is the step approach?

The stepwise approach to asthma is a description of the levels of treatment required to achieve good asthma control. If control at a particular step is not adequate, based on the above criteria, treatment must be increased to the next level or step. Sometimes it is necessary to move steps rapidly, or to miss out one or more steps. Once a patient's asthma is stable, he or she will probably remain at the therapeutic step that is successfully controlling the disease.

Patients should start at the step most appropriate for the initial severity of their condition. As asthma is a common inflammatory condition, most patients will need to receive anti-inflammatory drugs. Every patient should have a short-acting bronchodilator for relief of symptoms should they occur, but hopefully most will need to use it only rarely. Many patients will require a long-acting bronchodilator for symptom control as the third pillar of their asthma care.

Most patients' asthma will remain well controlled at the therapeutic step used to stabilize their disease and there will be no need to alter the steps over time.

A short course of oral steroids may be needed at any step should the asthma become unstable or be deteriorating more rapidly.

4.94 Where do I start?

When faced with a patient with probable or possible asthma, it can be difficult to decide on the best initial therapy for that patient. Start at the step most appropriate to the severity of the patient's asthma:

- *Step 1* – intermittent symptoms, less than once daily, no night symptoms, good lung function with little reversibility, no acute exacerbation in the last 12–18 months.
- *Step 2* – symptoms most days and occasional nights, lung function 60–80% of predicted value with some variability, or any acute exacerbation within the past 12–24 months irrespective of current or recent symptoms.
- *Step 3* – as for step 2, but daily symptoms and at night at least once a week; any severe exacerbation requiring admission, especially if needing intensive care or ventilation.

In practice, most people need to be at Step 2 or 3.

4.95 So what are the BTS/SIGN steps?

THE STEPS: ADULTS AND SCHOOLCHILDREN (5 YEARS AND OVER)

Step 1: Occasional use of bronchodilators
Inhaled short-acting β_2-agonists should be used to relieve symptoms as required rather than used regularly. If these drugs are needed more than two or three times a week on average, treatment should be stepped up.

Step 2: Regular inhaled steroids
Short-acting β_2-agonists as required *plus* inhaled beclometasone dipropionate or budesonide 200–800 µg daily or fluticasone propionate 200–400 µg daily. The lowest dose that maintains control should be used.

In an average general practice, the majority of asthmatics will be at this step for their chronic maintenance treatment.

Step 3: Regular use of inhaled steroids plus long-acting β_2-agonists
If the addition of long-acting β_2-agonists confers no benefit, consider trials of other add-on therapies.

Step 4: Inhaled steroids and long-acting β_2-agonists plus other agents
If the patient is stable but remains symptomatic despite regular inhaled

steroids plus inhaled long-acting β_2-agonists, the options are to add a sequential therapeutic trial of one or more of the following:

1 high-dose inhaled steroids (up to 2000 µg/day beclometasone or equivalent)
2 leukotriene receptor antagonists
3 sustained-release theophyllines
4 high-dose inhaled short-acting β_2-agonists
5 oral long-acting β_2-agonists
6 inhaled ipratropium or oxitropium
7 inhaled cromogens.

If there is no benefit from the addition of a new therapy after 2–4 weeks, stop it and substitute the next therapy. If there is partial benefit from a new therapy, continue it and add the next drug on the list.

■ High-dose inhaled short-acting β_2-agonists should be considered only if there has been an inadequate response to standard doses.
■ Increasing or decreasing the dose of inhaled steroids is no longer recommended as a routine option. If the asthma is well controlled on a particular dose, it makes sense to continue that dose, and to consider lowering the dose only when the asthma control is chronically stable and the patient is on high doses of inhaled steroids.
■ High-dose inhaled steroids should be used with caution in children and in patients more at risk from side-effects (e.g. diabetics, patients at risk of osteoporosis); be especially cautious about exceeding the manufacturer's maximum recommended doses and, if you do exceed them, discuss this fact with the patient and consider referral to a specialist.

Step 5: Addition of regular oral steroids
Step 5 therapy consists of the Step 4 therapy plus regular oral steroids in a single daily dose. The steps are summarized in *Fig. 4.1.*

THE STEPS: CHILDREN UNDER 5 YEARS OF AGE

Step 1
As for adults.

Step 2: Regular inhaled steroids
■ The addition of inhaled corticosteroids at 100–400 µg/day beclometasone or equivalent.
■ This should be used as first-line anti-inflammatory therapy.

Step 3: Inhaled steroids plus other agents, or higher-dose inhaled steroids
■ LTRAs can be tried in children aged 2 years or more.

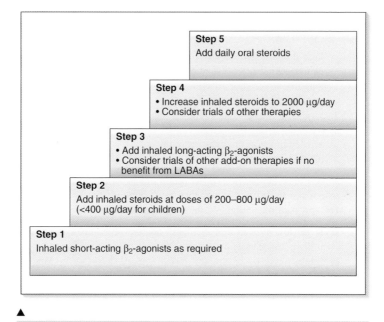

▲

Fig. 4.1 Summary of the BTS/SIGN steps. LABA, long-acting β_2-agonists.

■ Regular long-acting β_2-agonists can be added to the inhaled steroids if the asthma is triggered at night or by exercise in children aged 4 years and over.

■ High-dose inhaled steroids, up to 800 µg budesonide or beclometasone daily, or fluticasone 500 µg daily. If given by metered-dose inhalers, this should be via a large-volume spacer. Higher-dose inhaled steroids should be used with caution in all children, especially in those more at risk from side-effects (e.g. diabetics); be especially cautious about exceeding the manufacturer's maximum recommended doses and, if you do exceed them, discuss this fact with the patient's carer or parents.

Step 4: Higher-dose inhaled steroids plus other agents
High-dose inhaled steroids up to 800 µg a day, plus inhaled anticholinergics, or oral theophyllines (be mindful that there might be problems with safe and adequate doses in children) or oral long-acting bronchodilators if the patient cannot manage inhalers.

Step 5: Long-term oral steroids
Step 4 treatment plus regular oral prednisolone, ideally given on alternate days at the lowest effective dose.

Strongly consider sharing your management with a paediatrician before committing any child to Step 4 and, especially, Step 5 therapy.

4.96 What do I do if a patient has a short-term increase in symptoms?

Symptom relief is provided by using the reliever inhaler as often as needed (every 4 hours is the usually recommended interval). If the symptoms settle within a few days, this is the only treatment needed.

The emergence of night symptoms is more significant than having new, intermittent, daytime symptoms, but an increase in either should not be ignored and the asthma should be monitored (symptoms and peak flow) until stable again and for a further 48–96 hours afterwards. If the symptoms do not settle, or if they worsen, the patient should seek medical attention. A short course of oral steroids may be needed.

Telling patients to double their dose of inhaled steroids to cover any increase in symptoms or colds and other infections has been advocated for many years by many clinicians. There is no great evidence for the efficacy of this approach and it should be abandoned.

4.97 Do I have to go up and down the steps one at a time?

Most patients will not ever need to change steps. Some patients, however, may have experienced rapid deterioration in the past, and such patients should be advised to step up more than one step at a time. Thus, for example, a patient may be relatively well controlled on fairly low-dose inhaled steroids for nearly all of the year, but in response to an upper respiratory tract infection the asthma rapidly deteriorates. In the past this may have led to emergency hospital admission. Such patients may need to double or treble their dose of inhaled steroid and regularly take inhaled bronchodilators. Some patients will also benefit from taking short courses of oral steroids as soon as their peak flow deteriorates or symptoms increase.

4.98 When should a patient come back down from a temporary high step?

Once a patient has stepped up their treatment, they should remain on the higher doses until the symptoms have abated and their peak flow has returned to normal with little or no variability. They should wait a further 48–96 hours before reducing back to their previous level. If they have increased by two or more steps, they can reduce back down to their maintenance level without having to step down through each of the intervening steps. The reason for the temporary poor control must be elicited and addressed. If there is no clear reason, or if episodes of poor control occur several times a year, do not step down, but maintain at the higher step (*See Q. 4.101*).

4.99 What do I do if the patient doesn't respond?

Oral steroids should be recommended as step-up therapy for anybody who has previously had sudden or severe deterioration in their previously well-controlled asthma, or if their control is poor and failing to respond to an increase in treatment step or steps. Oral steroids are also necessary for patients who are already on Step 4 treatment for maintenance therapy.

4.100 When should I step up long-term therapy?

If a patient's asthma is imperfectly controlled over several weeks or months, or they need temporarily to increase their treatment at regular or frequent intervals, they should step up their chronic therapy to the next appropriate level. The following indicates that the chronic maintenance therapy is inadequate, and the patient should step up their treatment:

- Any acute severe exacerbation needing hospitalization, especially if admitted for more than 24 hours, or admitted to intensive care, or ventilated.
- Frequent symptoms (most days or 1–2 times per week during the night) especially if episodic and recurrent.
- Any need for more than one course of oral steroids in the previous 6–12 months.
- Asthma that results in impaired functioning (poor exercise tolerance, time off work or school, any disability).

4.101 When should I step down long-term therapy?

This is a difficult question to answer because there has not been a great deal of published evidence to help us. It is important to try to achieve the best possible control of a patient's asthma, all the time. The emphasis on stepping down is less than previously advised, and it is better to risk overtreatment than to risk deterioration in long-term asthma control.

Before stepping down, patients should be symptom-free (including sleeping through the night and having appropriate exercise tolerance), with stable peak flow readings and needing to use their relieving inhalers rarely (less than twice a week) or not at all. They should not have had an exacerbation needing oral steroids or high-dose bronchodilators for at least 12 months, and not had an exacerbation needing emergency visits by the GP or to hospital in the last 24 months. If they have needed hospital admission for acute severe asthma, and especially if they needed ventilation or admission to intensive care, be very wary of ever stepping down and consider an even longer period of stability if you and the patient do decide to step down therapy. Be especially wary of stepping down from regular use of inhaled steroids: there are few adults for whom this should be advocated. Stopping inhaled steroids removes all anti-inflammatory protection from the airways and can result in severe sudden asthma or in chronic low-grade symptoms and subtle unnecessary diminution in quality of life.

In children, these periods can be reduced quite substantially; the younger the child, the shorter the interval. Again, be cautious when contemplating removal of the protection of inhaled steroids. However, there are no clear rules or guidelines.

4.102 Why should I step down?

One of the concepts of all preventive medicine is that the patient should be on the minimum treatment necessary to control the disease. This principle is valid for asthma.

ECONOMIC REASONS

The most important reason is economic. It is extravagant for patients to take more medication than they need to control their disease. In asthma, higher-dose inhaled steroids and all long-acting β_2-agonists and LTRAs are relatively expensive, so reducing the dose to the minimum needed will be less expensive for the health service.

> ### Side effects
> With the exeption of the LTRAs, which are relatively free from side-effects, oral medication used to manage asthma is more likely to cause dose-related side-effects than inhaled medications. Stopping or reducing oral medication is usually the first reduction recommended when stepping down. Asthma patients are extremely unlikely to suffer or risk dose-related side-effects from inhaled medication at or below the doses recommended by the manufacturers, so there is less compelling need to step down from the point of view of drug safety.

4.103 Does it matter if I step down too slowly or too quickly?

Too slowly: no, unless the patient is suffering from side-effects.
Too quickly: yes, the patient's condition is more likely to deteriorate and an acute exacerbation may occur. If oral steroids are reduced or stopped inappropriately, patients are at risk of adrenocortical insufficiency, with potentially fatal consequences.

SELF-MANAGEMENT PLANS

4.104 What is a self-management plan?

The current model usually employed is to empower the asthmatic to alter their therapy in certain circumstances. The asthmatic (or parent) then needs to know what to do, how to do it, and what to do if the exacerbation does or does not get better. This implies that the patient is aware of worsening asthma by being able to:

■ Recognize the symptoms.
■ Realize the implications of increased need for relievers.
■ Objectively measure the deterioration.

Self-management plans include simple action plans like the three points above, and are sufficient for the majority of patients with mild to moderate asthma (Steps 1–3) who are managed in primary care. More detailed self-management plans may be needed for a minority of patients whose asthma is or has been unstable or very severe.

These asthma management plans give control to the asthmatic. This control can be used effectively only if the asthmatic has received sufficient

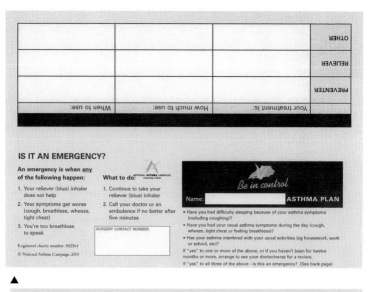

▲

Fig. 4.2 A Personal Action Plan for use by anyone who has asthma, particularly if it is mild to moderate. This is folded in half lengthways, then in half again to become credit card-sized. By kind permission of the National Asthma Campaign.

SWINDON ASTHMA GROUP

Asthma Self Management Plan

		Best ever peak flow:		Any allergies:		
Treatment Level	Symptoms	Peak flow	Drug	Device	Dose	Frequency
1. Maintenance	WELL	Over	1.			
	• no night symptoms		2.			
	• no day symptoms	....	3.			
	• no exercise limitations		4.			
2. Step up	UNWELL	Between	1.			
	• night cough or wheeze		2.			
	• day cough or wheeze	....	3.			
	• exercise symptoms	and	4.			
	• need for more reliever		5.			
	• cold or other illness	....	6.			
3. Severe	VERY UNWELL	Less than	1.			
	• any of the above worse despite step up treatment		2.			
		....	3.			
			4.			
	• reliever not working as well or as long as usual		5.			
			6.			
			AND INFORM YOUR GP/PRACTICE NURSE THAT DAY			

IF YOU ARE RAPIDLY GETTING WORSE OR IF YOU CANNOT TALK OR EAT AND YOU CANNOT CONTACT YOUR GP IN AN EMERGENCY, GO TO THE NEAREST HOSPITAL ACCIDENT AND EMERGENCY DEPARTMENT- DIAL 999 IF NECESSARY

Relievers:	1.	2.	3.	4.	(Take just when needed)
Preventers/protectors	1.	2.	3.	4.	(Take regularly)

Your Name:	Your GP's Name:
D O B:	Address:
Address:	
Telephone:	Telephone:

If you attend a hospital:	
Hospital Name:	
Address:	
Telephone:	Unit Number:
Consultant	

If you have increased your treatment, stay on the step up or severe level until you are feeling well again and your peak flow is over......and for a further 2 days, then reduce to your maintenance level.

▲

Fig. 4.3 A more complex self-management plan for use by patients who have unstable or severe chronic asthma.

education, training and monitoring, and is compliant with treatment and can use inhalers correctly. The management plans need to be tailored for each asthmatic and to be negotiated and agreed by each asthmatic and their professional carers. The plans need to be written down; both parties should keep a copy. Each plan should be reviewed at least annually and after each exacerbation to see whether it was as effective as possible. Examples of self-management plans are included in *Figs 4.2 and 4.3*.

Temporary increases in treatment are also recommended to cover periods of increased risk of deterioration, such as during colds or other infections, and also to cover periods of travel or being away from home. The higher levels of treatment should ideally be started before exposure and continued for 2–3 days after the exposure is over.

4.105 Do self-management plans really help?

There is increasing objective evidence for the benefit of this type of asthma management. Self-management plans for patients with asthma reduce hospital admission rates for asthma and also the amount of income lost by patients because of illness. A symptom-based asthma self-management plan results in fewer days off work, fewer night symptoms, fewer acute exacerbations and increased mean peak flow readings. Studies have shown that patients randomized to having a self-management plan showed decreased hospital admissions, decreased consultation with asthma symptoms, decreased courses of oral steroids, and decreased emergency nebulizations compared with patients who did not receive a self-management plan.[31] However, despite randomization, measures of patient morbidity in the intervention group before the issue of self-management plans were much higher than in the control group. This was probably because GPs in the intervention group issued self-management plans to patients with poorly controlled asthma rather than to all patients who were eligible to receive them.

A further randomized trial[32] of guided self-management plans against traditional treatment did not show this 'enthusiast bias'. This trial showed that the introduction of self-management plans reduced the incidence of acute exacerbations and symptoms and increased the quality of life of the asthmatics. Whether this improvement was due purely to the introduction of self-management plans or whether it also included changes due to the early treatment of airway inflammation, and patient education about asthma and improved general compliance with treatment, is not clear.

It therefore seems sensible to ensure that all patients with asthma have both verbal and written advice about asthma, with the advice tailored for each individual. Detailed self-management plans and peak flow meters should be given, as a minimum, to adults with severe asthma, to those with variable disease and to those who have been admitted to hospital because of asthma. Whether details of self-management plans, especially those that are peak flow led, should be given to all other groups of asthmatics is still unclear.

4.106 How can patients recognize deterioration?

There are three ways of recognizing deteriorating asthma. Every asthmatic should be instructed and educated about each of them:

■ An increase in the symptoms of cough, wheeze, chest tightness and shortness of breath, especially at night, or a decrease in exercise tolerance, should alert the asthmatic to the need for increased medication and increased surveillance.
■ If symptom control can be maintained only by using more relieving drugs, especially if the drugs seem to work less well or for less time.
■ Finally, peak flow readings provide an excellent objective measurement of airway obstruction. A change in symptoms or need for relieving treatment should certainly be an indication for all asthmatics to start twice-daily peak flow reading until the levels are consistently normal again.

See also Q. 2.15.

4.107 Should all patients measure their peak flow every day?

It is probably unreasonable for most patients to be measuring their peak flow twice daily continuously, but they should certainly do so in the circumstances mentioned in *Q. 4.99–4.103*, as well as when treatment has been altered, they have a cold or other infection, or are going to be or have been exposed to a known trigger (such as staying in a house with pets).

Patients with moderate to severe asthma should measure their peak flow regularly all the time.

Patients who have unstable or difficult to control asthma, or those who have sudden, very severe episodes, should also measure their peak flow regularly (ideally twice a day, every day).

4.108 How can patients know what to do if they think their asthma is getting worse?

They will need to be properly instructed by their doctor or nurse. This should be part of the education of all asthmatics and their carers. They will need to know:

■ How and when they can recognize that their asthma is getting worse.
■ What they should do to try to make their asthma better again.
■ How and when they need to call for help because the measures they have taken have been inadequate.

4.109 What should patients do if they think their asthma is deteriorating?

■ Use their bronchodilator inhaler regularly: 2–4 puffs every 3–4 hours.
■ Monitor their peak flow and symptoms.
■ Double their inhaled steroid dose if they have found this helpful in the past; otherwise of doubtful value.

4.110 So what peak flow levels are important?

For a given peak flow reduction, the patient needs to know how to increase the medication:

■ At levels above 70% of predicted, continue the chronic medication.
■ At levels between 50% and 70% use the reliever medication regularly every 4 hours or so, and continue monitoring the peak flow.
■ If the peak flow returns to that predicted, stay on the higher levels of therapy for a further two days.

See also Q. 2.15, Q. 2.17 and Q. 2.18.

4.111 When should patients call for help?

■ If peak flow falls to below 50%.
■ If peak flow does not improve after a few days.
■ If the symptoms are not improving after 24–48 hours.
■ If the symptoms are getting worse (decreased exercise tolerance, inability to talk freely, difficulty dressing or eating).
■ If there are unusual symptoms (haemoptysis, fever).
■ If the patient or carer is worried.

Patients should seek medical help that day.

4.112 Which patients should have access to home oral steroids?

■ Short-course oral steroid therapy may be needed to prevent or terminate exacerbations.
■ Asthmatics who experience sudden severe exacerbations in response to certain triggers, such as colds or allergen exposure, may benefit from prompt oral steroid use before or as soon as possible after exposure, so should have access to home oral steroids.
■ Some patients who use complex, written, self-management plans may need home steroids as part of their plan. These patients will tend to have more severe asthma.

4.113 What type of steroid tablets should they have?

- ■ The first dose should not be enteric-coated tablets as their absorption may be slow and unpredictable.
- ■ Subsequent doses are usually given as enteric-coated preparations, which may reduce gastric irritation.
- ■ Children require soluble tablets (steroid syrups or medicine are not available in the UK).
- ■ The complete daily dose should be taken at one time, preferably in the morning to avoid sleep disturbance and to minimize adrenal suppression.
- ■ There is no need to diminish the dose gradually if courses last less than three weeks.

4.114 When should patients start their home steroids?

Some asthmatics may have oral steroids at home and these should be started while waiting to see the doctor or nurse if the peak flow has fallen to 50% the predicted value (75 L/min in children under 8 years old). This advice is also recommended if any asthmatic has very severe symptoms that are not relieved promptly by the increased treatment.

The threshold for using oral steroids varies with each asthmatic. Those whose exacerbations have previously been sudden or severe should take them at a very early stage, sometimes with only a 20% drop in peak flow or with the first symptoms of deterioration.

Oral steroids should be started at agreed points in the self-management plan, usually when the peak flow has fallen to 50% of best ever, or the symptoms are worsening rapidly or declining despite regular bronchodilator use.

When taking oral steroids asthmatics should monitor their peak flow and continue on the steroids until the peak flow is consistently normal, and then for at least a further two days.

Emergency care should be sought, either from the GP or, if not available, from the local accident and emergency department.

4.115 Should self-management plans be symptom or peak flow led?

Most patients prefer management plans that are based both on symptoms and peak flow.

The use of symptom-only self-management plans appears to be sufficient for most patients, but many asthmatics are poor discriminators of just how severe their asthma is. In other words, they cannot interpret the severity of their asthma solely from their symptoms. Overall, it is clear that management plans do work. It is also becoming increasingly clear that the peak flow is not always the crucial ingredient. Teaching the asthmatic the importance of changes of their symptoms, and the appropriate action to be taken when a deterioration occurs, are the keys to successful asthma management. Prescribing a peak flow meter without a guided self-management plan and regular review is of no use.

4.116 Are there any examples I can use?

Figs 4.2 and 4.3 show two examples of written self-management plans. The Swindon Asthma Group plan (*Fig. 4.3*) is detailed and quite complex, but is useful for patients with severe unstable asthma. The National Asthma Campaign's self-management plan (*Fig. 4.2*) is simpler and easier, but offers less flexibility.

Most patients do not need such detailed plans, but benefit from a simple Action Plan such as:

1   If you think your asthma is worse, take your blue puffer every 4 hours until you feel your asthma is back to normal, and for a further two days.
2   If your asthma gets even worse, or is not back to your normal within 2–3 days, see your doctor or nurse.
3   If your asthma is getting rapidly worse, see your doctor or nurse as soon as you can.
4   Go to the emergency department at your hospital if you can't contact your doctor or nurse.

ACUTE ASTHMA

4.117 How can I recognize acute severe asthma?

Features of severe asthma include:
■ Difficulty completing a sentence in a single breath
■ Respiratory rate of over 25 per minute
■ Heart rate of over 110 per minute
■ Peak flow of less than 50% of best ever or predicted.

Life-threatening features are:

■ Peak flow of less than 33% of best ever or predicted
■ Cyanosis
■ Bradycardia, hypotension
■ Silent chest
■ Confusion, exhaustion or coma.

In children, features of severe asthma are:

- Child too breathless to talk or feed
- Respiratory rate of over 50 per minute, heart rate of over 140 per minute
- Peak flow of less than 50% best ever.

Life-threatening features are:

- Peak flow of less than 33% best ever
- Silent chest
- Cyanosis, fatigue, exhaustion, agitation and altered levels of consciousness.

In infants there may be associated dehydration and vomiting. Treatment should be maximal and prompt.

Assessment is by:

- History
- Examination
- Peak flow measurement, if at all possible.

4.118 What about acute asthma – which drugs do I use first?

OXYGEN

- Give oxygen at high flows and high concentrations continuously until improvement has occurred and been maintained.
- Carbon dioxide retention is not aggravated by oxygen therapy in asthma.
- Patients die from hypoxia in acute asthma; oxygen is crucial to preventing death in severe acute asthma.

INHALED β_2-AGONISTS

- A large-volume spacer with sequential actuations of 20 puffs of a β_2-agonist is as effective as nebulized β_2-agonists.
- If a nebulizer is used, use oxygen to drive the nebulizer if possible.
- Use salbutamol (albuterol) 2.5–5 mg or terbutaline 5–10 mg (half-doses for children).

SYSTEMIC STEROIDS

- Give oral prednisolone 30–60 mg in one dose (children 2 mg/kg).
- Use soluble prednisolone for children.
- Do not use enteric-coated prednisolone for the first dose as this delays absorption.
- If the patient is vomiting or unable to take oral medication, give intravenous hydrocortisone at 100–200 mg in adults and 4 mg/kg in children.

IPRATROPIUM BROMIDE

■ This is best reserved for those asthmatics who deteriorate or fail to improve rapidly when treated with the standard regimen of oxygen, steroids and β_2-agonists.

■ Patients who benefit most from the addition of ipratropium to salbutamol (albuterol) are those who have received relatively little inhaled β_2-agonists before presentation – not necessarily those with the most severe asthma.

■ There are some doubts about the clinical efficacy of adding ipratropium bromide to salbutamol (albuterol) in acute childhood asthma, but there are fewer doubts about the efficacy of the combination in acute adult asthma.

AMINOPHYLLINE

Intravenous aminophylline can be given in addition to high-dose bronchodilators, high-dose oral or intravenous steroids and oxygen. Its use is best reserved for patients with severe life-threatening asthma that is responding inadequately to treatment with oxygen, steroids and high-dose β_2-agonist.

Particular care must be used in giving intravenous aminophylline to patients who are taking long-term oral theophyllines, especially if they also have a viral infection as it can be difficult to avoid a toxic dose.

> Intravenous aminophylline produces serious side-effects, mainly cardiac dysrhythmias that can be fatal. It should only be given under electrocardiographic control.

4.119 If the patient responds, what do I do next?

■ If clinical improvement follows and the peak flow increases to a minimum of 50% predicted and has improved by at least 20% from pretreatment levels, advise 4-hourly high-dose inhaled β_2-agonists, continue high-dose oral steroids taken as one dose each morning, and continue maintenance therapy at the dose indicated by the peak flow management plan or at double the usual dose.

■ Review after 4 hours or so.

■ Ensure the asthmatic has a peak flow meter which they can use correctly, and ensure they use it to monitor their progress every 4 hours or so.

■ Ensure they have clear, written instruction on how to recognize further deterioration and how and when to get further medical help.

■ If improvement is maintained, arrange further follow-up and review.

■ Stop oral steroids once the peak flow has remained stable and at best-ever or predicted levels for at least two days.

4.120 What if the patient doesn't respond – what do I do then?

If clinical improvement is inadequate, or the peak flow is still less than 50% predicted or has not improved by at least 20%, arrange immediate hospital admission. Be sure to inform the ambulance service that you require an urgent ambulance, with a crew able to administer oxygen and nebulizer therapy. Nebulized salbutamol (albuterol) has been shown to be effective and safe in acute asthma when administered by ambulance personnel who have had a short training course.

While waiting for the ambulance, repeat the nebulized or inhaled agent via spacer bronchodilators. If further deterioration occurs, give subcutaneous bronchodilators: salbutamol 250–500 μg (children 5 μg/kg) or terbutaline 250–500 μg (children 10 μg/kg) or 1:1000 adrenaline 0.5 mL.

If further deterioration occurs give intravenous bronchodilators: aminophylline 250 mg over 30 minutes (if not already on theophyllines) (children 5 μg/kg) or salbutamol 4 μg/kg over 10 minutes (not recommended for children) or terbutaline 250 μg over 10 minutes (children over the age of 12, 10 μg/kg).

Do not give sedatives, antibiotics (unless clinically indicated) or physiotherapy.

Admission is also advised, although not necessarily via an emergency ambulance:

■ If the asthmatic and/or their carers cannot cope safely with assessing the severity of the attack or cannot cope with adjusting the treatment
■ If the asthmatic has no access to a telephone or they are remote from sources of help.

A lower threshold for admission is appropriate in patients:

■ Seen in the latter part of the day
■ With recently worsening symptoms
■ With recent onset of night symptoms
■ Who have had previous severe attacks, especially if they then deteriorated rapidly.

4.121 What about follow-up after an episode of acute asthma – when should I see the patient and what should I do?

After every acute exacerbation, follow-up should always be arranged. The patient should be seen about 4–6 hours after the acute episode, and then 2–3 days later. The patient should be clear when and how to call for help before then, should the asthma deteriorate. The trigger for the exacerbation should be identified, if possible, and advice given on possible future avoidance. The self-management plan should be reviewed or instigated. Adjustment to the plan may be needed, especially the criteria for when and how to call for help. It may be worth advising on the use of oral steroids at an earlier stage of deterioration, or even prophylactically if exposure to similar triggers is unavoidable in the future. Obviously such patients should be prescribed a supply of oral steroids with reinforcing written instructions on when to start them, the dose, and when to stop them.

In small children or adults unable to use a peak flow meter, assessment will have to be solely on clinical grounds, so more frequent reviews, especially initially, need to be made.

INHALER DEVICES

4.122 What types of inhaler device are there?

There is an increasing variety of devices through which asthma drugs can be given. The increasing number of these devices, and which ones are available for the delivery of which drugs, causes some confusion to patients and clinicians alike (*see Appendix B*).

An inhaler is a device that delivers a drug by inhalation. 'Inhaler' is a collective term for all the devices used in the management of asthma, which are listed in *Appendix B*, as well as including nebulizers and large-volume spacers (*see also Chs 5 and 6*). The wide range of inhaler devices available allows treatment to be tailored to individual patient's needs, abilities and preferences.

The following categories of inhaler device are available:

■ *Metered-dose aerosols*. These are specific, propellant-driven devices. They may be used alone or with spacers.
■ *Breath-actuated devices*. The dose of drug is released when the device is triggered by the patient inspiring through the device.
■ *Dry powder devices*. The dose of drug is in a powder which is inhaled through the device.
■ *Nebulizers*. These are powered machines that disperse the dose of drug into a fine mist, which can then be inhaled.

4.123 How do I decide which inhaler device to recommend?

In treating asthma, care in explaining and demonstrating inhaler technique may be more important than the choice of drugs in a particular category.

> The correct choice of device and proper teaching of its use can be fundamental in determining the level of success in treating asthma.

When choosing a device, choose *with* the patient. Patients will only use devices that they are able to use and which they like. The device must be able to give trouble-free treatment reliably, consistently, easily and conveniently. The size, shape and weight may be important to some patients. Remember that a patient's treatment may be life-saving, so it is essential that each patient is able to use their inhaler easily and reliably, even when stressed and breathless and capable of only low inspiratory flows.

- Some patients lack the manual dexterity or visual acuity needed to operate some devices correctly.
- Peer pressure and local fashion may be important in device selection, especially for children and teenagers.
- The most expensive device is the one the patient doesn't use.

Preparations available as MDIs are shown in *Appendix C*.

METERED-DOSE INHALERS

4.124 What are the advantages and disadvantages of metered-dose inhalers?

This is the 'universal' inhaler, often known simply as the 'aerosol inhaler' or 'metered-dose inhaler' (the MDI).

The MDI is a small pressurized canister that sits in a plastic device. When the canister is pressed into the device, a metered amount of aerosol is released from the canister through a small tube that fits into the patient's mouth. Examples are shown in *Fig. 4.4*.

Deposition in the lungs with perfect technique is about 10–15% of the dose delivered by the aerosol.

Advantages of MDIs include:

- Compact and portable
- Easy for some people to use

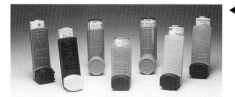

◀ **Fig. 4.4** Some examples of metered-dose inhalers. Photograph by kind permission of Ivax Pharmaceuticals UK Ltd.

- Require no preparation except shaking
- Quick and unobtrusive
- Nearly all inhaled drugs are available as MDIs even if they come as other inhalers as well
- Usually the cheapest form available of most drugs.

Disadvantages of MDIs include:

- Not all patients can use MDIs adequately – overall about 50% of asthmatic patients cannot use an MDI properly.
- Some patients stop inhaling when the cold propellant reaches the back of the mouth – the 'cold freon' effect.
- There is no means of telling the number of doses used or remaining, and so it can sometimes be difficult to know when the canister is empty, except by judging its weight or shaking it to hear the splash of fluid within the canister.

> It cannot be overemphasized that, unless a metered-dose inhaler is used correctly, the patient will not get the full dose of the relevant drug and will therefore not derive the full benefit from the drug, which has been imperfectly delivered.

4.125 How do you use a MDI?

Shake the device vigorously for 10–20 seconds. Remove the outer cap from the device, inhale deeply, then exhale fully. Put your lips firmly around the mouthpiece of the device, keeping the device upright all the time. Breathe in slowly and, as soon as you start to breathe in, press down firmly on the aerosol canister in the device; continue breathing in slowly and deeply to full inspiration. Hold your breath as long as you can, remove the device from your mouth, and then exhale. Get you breath back, then repeat the whole process (including shaking the device again for 10–20 seconds) for each subsequent dose.

4.126 Should I replace all my patients' CFC-driven inhalers with HFA-driven ones?

MDIs are propellant driven, and the propellant currently contains chlorofluorocarbons (CFCs) in most of the available inhalers. Replacement CFC-free MDIs will be increasingly introduced over the next few years. The CFC is replaced by hydrofluoroalkane (HFA) propellants. The reason for the change is not pharmacological but environmental, as part of the worldwide agreements on reducing CFC use. It is important that patients are maintained on their current MDI until that product is available in a

CFC-free form. Switching should not be made without consulting with the patient and making sure that they are in agreement.

4.127 Are there any differences in CFC- and HFA-driven inhalers? Which do patients prefer?

In terms of efficacy, there are no differences between the two. HFA-driven MDIs may actually increase lung deposition as the particle size of the drug in the aerosol spray is smaller, allowing the spray to travel more distally into the airways and increasing the distribution over a larger area of airway mucosa.

The aerosol spray undoubtedly tastes different and the canister will feel different when HFA propellants rather than CFC propellants are used, but most patients soon get used to the new taste and feel.

The nozzle on the aerosol canister may get blocked more easily and patients should check the nozzle occasionally. If it is even partially blocked, the nozzle of the aerosol canister should be rinsed in warm water and allowed to air dry.

Patients may be resistant to changing their inhaler from a CFC- to a HFA-driven one, but, if forewarned and told about the advantages to the environment, very few patients are unable to adapt within a few days. The vast majority of patients can be happily and successfully switched to HFA-driven inhalers.

SPACERS

4.128 What about spacers – what types are there?

Spacer devices attach to MDIs and act as a reservoir from which the drug can be inhaled, making good coordination of the MDI actuation with inspiration less critical.

The important difference is that the aerosol cloud produced from spacer devices is finer and slower moving than when given from a MDI alone. Spacers can therefore increase the amount of drug reaching the lower airways and reduce impaction of the drug in the mouth and throat. They are thus particularly useful for giving inhaled steroids because they can help to reduce the risk of local systemic side-effects. At least 20% of the dose delivered by the aerosol will be delivered to the lungs via the spacer.

There are three main types of spacer: large-, medium- and small-volume spacers.

LARGE-VOLUME SPACERS

- Have a volume of about 750 mL.
- Have a one-way valve in the mouthpiece. The valve spacer devices serve as a holding chamber for the aerosol and eliminate the need to

coordinate inhalation with actuation, enabling the patient to inhale the dose over several breaths if necessary.

■ Tend to be the most effective but also the most cumbersome.

■ Examples include the Volumatic (see *Fig. 4.5* on p. 147) and the Nebuhaler.

MEDIUM-VOLUME SPACERS

■ Have a volume of 100–350 mL.

■ Examples include the AeroChamber, Babyhaler and NebuChamber.

SMALL-VOLUME SPACERS

■ Have a volume of about 10–50 mL.

■ Are basically an open tube device in which the metered-dose aerosol is fired into a reservoir; some synchronized inhalation is still required.

■ Examples include the Optimiser and Spacehaler, which are used with MDIs. The Rotahaler and Spinhaler are used with dry powdered preparations.

There are important differences in the outputs from different inhalers used with different spacers. Ideally one should use the spacer only with the designated inhaler, which usually means that the spacer and the inhalers are made by the same company. Licensing and use should be restricted to specified combinations of drug and spacers.

4.129 What are the advantages and disadvantages of spacers?

ADVANTAGES

■ Easy to use.

■ Suitable for all ages.

■ Relatively cheap.

■ Increase the fraction of the dose of drug delivered to the lung and decrease the fraction of drug deposited in the mouth and throat.

■ Improve the pulmonary bioavailability of drugs in normal volunteers who could use a MDI correctly.

■ Can be used as a substitute for a nebulizer in acute asthma if sufficient doses are released into the chamber; about 20 doses of a bronchodilator given one puff at a time is usually adequate.

■ Provide a cheaper way of giving effective treatment especially if high-dose inhaled steroids are required. High-dose fluticasone given via a spacer and MDI is at least as effective as nebulized budesonide, while costing about half the price – and being quicker and easier for patients to use.

■ More importantly, they can also help to reduce the risk of local and systemic side-effects because of reduced oropharyngeal deposition.

DISADVANTAGES

■ Bulky and obtrusive, especially the large-volume spacers
■ Need to ensure that the MDI fits the spacer correctly.

4.130 Which spacer should I recommend?

Generally, large-volume spacers are the most efficient but the most bulky; medium-volume spacers are more portable and a little less efficient; and small-volume spacers are very much less efficient although very portable and convenient.

LARGE-VOLUME SPACERS

The Volumatic is designed for all Allen & Hanbury inhalers, which include Ventolin, Becotide, Becloforte, Flixotide, Serevent and Ventide. The Nebuhaler is designed for all Astra MDIs, which include Bricanyl and Pulmicort. The Fisonair is designed for use with Intal, but its port will loosely fit other MDIs. All three spacers have a capacity of at least 700 mL.

MEDIUM-VOLUME SPACERS

The AeroChamber is a medium-sized spacer with a one-way diaphragm valve of low resistance. It comes with either a mouthpiece or a mask for adults. It is also available as a child's device with a mask, and as an infant's device with a mask. It has a universal port which holds any MDI very snugly. The Babyhaler has a soft face mask and small volume, so is emptied by far fewer breaths, even by small babies, and contains inlet and outlet valves that operate at very low flow rates. The NebuChamber is a medium-sized metal spacer to which a face mask may be attached. It is made from stainless steel, so is non-electrostatic, has a very small dead space and very low pressure valves.

The medium-volume spacers have volumes between 80 and 300 mL.

SMALL-VOLUME SPACERS

The Optimiser is a small-volume spacer available for use with the Easi-Breathe breath-actuated MDIs. By reducing the velocity of the flow of the aerosol spray, the cold freon effect is reduced. The amount of drug deposited in the mouth and throat is also reduced, as well as improving the amount reaching the lungs. The Spacehaler greatly reduces the velocity of the aerosol cloud that emerges from the MDI, so increasing the respirable fraction of the drug delivered to the patient. It can be as effective as using a large-volume spacer. The Space Inhaler is available with Astra MDIs (terbutaline and budesonide) and has similar properties to the other small-volume spacers. The Syncroner is a small-volume spacer that is available as an integral unit with Intal (cromoglycate), Tilade (nedocromil) or Aerocrom (salbutamol–cromoglycate) MDIs.

The small-volume spacers have volumes of less than 30 mL.

Finally, if there is no spacer available, one can improvise by using a polystyrene cup. The metered-dose aerosol mouthpiece can be pushed through the bottom of the polystyrene cup, and the cup placed over an infant's face to act as a small-volume spacer for emergency use.

4.131 How should patients use spacers?

The technique of inhaling from a spacer is the same, irrespective of the type or size of the spacer:

1 Shake the MDI and remove its cap.
2 Insert spacer into the relevant port of the spacer.
3 Put the spacer into the mouth.
4 Actuate the MDI once.
5 Inhale as deeply as possible, holding the breath for as long as comfortable at full inspiration.
6 Remove spacer from the mouth and exhale.
7 Remove MDI from the spacer and repeat the whole process for the second and any subsequent puffs.

An alternative at Stage 5 is to take six tidal breaths through the spacer. This is especially useful for patients unable to inhale deeply or to hold their breath for long and for large-volume spacers.

Whichever technique is used, the aim is to keep the time between actuation of the MDI and full inspiration as short as possible.

4.132 Do patients need to care for their spacers?

The spacer manufacturers recommend that patients change their spacers every year, although, in practice, few patients actually do so.

All spacers should be cleaned once a week or so by washing in weak washing-up liquid solution, rinsing and allowing the spacer to air dry.

4.133 What about spacers in children with asthma?

In small children and babies, the large-volume spacers can be used with the addition of the soft face mask that fits over the mouthpiece; this forms a seal around the child's face. Babies and toddlers do not have sufficient inspiratory flow to move the valve on the device. The MDI is actuated as before, and the child is held firmly either between the knees or as if about to give the child a bottle. The mask is then placed firmly over the child's nose and, if the whole device is tilted upwards from the vertical, the valve falls open and the child just needs to breathe entirely normally and cannot but help inhaling the contents of the spacer, as shown in *Fig. 4.5*. About 6–10 breaths are required from small children to empty the spacer completely. It

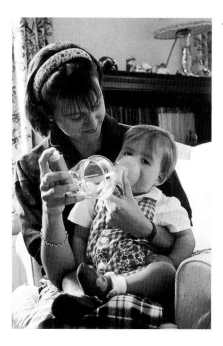

Fig. 4.5 A large-volume spacer such as the Volumatic is an efficient method of delivering inhaled therapy, especially if the patient cannot use a metered-dose inhaler. Its use with a small child is illustrated here.

is obviously undesirable, but should the child cry, the lung deposition is still acceptable.

BREATH-ACTUATED DEVICES

4.134 What are breath-actuated devices?

Breath-actuated devices are aerosols that are actuated by the patient's own inspiration rather than relying on a pressurized propellant. They are metered-dose inhalers that have been adapted so that the patient does not need to coordinate actuation of the inhaler with respiration. Two types are currently available: the Easi-Breathe (*Fig. 4.6*) and the Autohaler (*Fig. 4.7*). The devices need to be primed first, either by opening the cap, as for the Easi-Breathe, or by lifting a lever on top of the device, as for the Autohaler. The dose is then released automatically when the patient breathes in through the mouthpiece.

4.135 How do patients use breath-actuated aerosols?

The device should be gently shaken for several seconds and the protective cap removed. The patient breathes in fully then breathes out fully. The

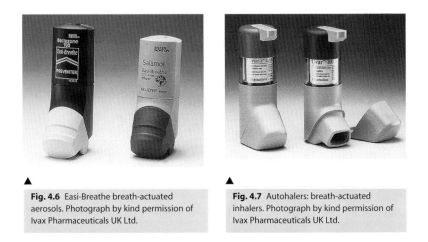

▲

Fig. 4.6 Easi-Breathe breath-actuated aerosols. Photograph by kind permission of Ivax Pharmaceuticals UK Ltd.

▲

Fig. 4.7 Autohalers: breath-actuated inhalers. Photograph by kind permission of Ivax Pharmaceuticals UK Ltd.

patient places their lips firmly around the mouthpiece and inhales as deeply as possible. The breath should be held for as long as possible, and the inhaler removed from the mouth. The patient then exhales. If further doses are required the inhaler should be shaken again and the patient should be breathing comfortably before attempting a further inhalation.

4.136 What are the advantages and disadvantages of breath-actuated aerosols?

ADVANTAGES

There is no need to synchronize actuation with inhalation. They are therefore very easy to use by people of all ages. Other advantages are as for the conventional metered-dose aerosol. The Easi-Breathe has an integral cap which, therefore, cannot get lost or be inhaled inadvertently.

DISADVANTAGES

There is no means of counting doses, so patients can find it difficult to know when the inhaler is nearly empty. Breath-actuated aerosols are larger and heavier than the conventional metered-dose aerosol, and some are relatively more expensive. Oropharyngeal deposition is similar to, or slightly more than, that with metered-dose aerosols. Some breath-actuated devices make a sharp click during actuation, which can be alarming especially for children, and as a result they may stop inhaling.

DRY POWDERED DEVICES

4.137 What are dry powdered devices?

Dry powdered devices are breath actuated. They rely on the patient's own inspiration to dispose the drug powder into an aerosol of drug particles, which is then inhaled into the lungs. They contain the active drug either alone or combined with powder. This powder is usually lactose, the taste of which can help patients tell whether they have inhaled the dose (this is safe for diabetics). They fall into two main categories: devices that are preloaded and those that require loading.

Preloaded devices include the Accuhaler (*Fig. 4.8*), the Pulvinal, the Twisthaler, the Turbohaler or Turbuhaler (*Fig. 4.9*) and the Clickhaler.

Devices that require loading include the Aerohaler, the Aerolizer, the Diskhaler (Diskus), the Novolizer and the Spinhaler. In some of these devices the drug and powder is in a single capsule that needs to be loaded individually into the device before the patient uses it, such as the Rotahaler, Spinhaler or Aerolizer. The Diskhaler is used with a disc containing 4–8 doses of drug; the disc needs to be changed at the end of the number of doses. The Aerohaler has a drum that can be loaded with six capsules before use. The cartridge is not replaced, but just reloaded with another six capsules.

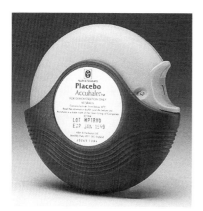

▲

Fig. 4.8 The Accuhaler is a dry powder device that does not require preloading. Photograph by kind permission of Ivax Pharmaceuticals UK Ltd.

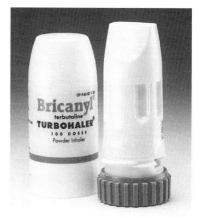

▲

Fig. 4.9 Turbohaler: an example of a dry powder device that does not require preloading. Photograph by kind permission of Ivax Pharmaceuticals UK Ltd.

The Novolizer has a cartridge containing 100 or 200 doses of drug, which is replaced when empty.

4.138 How do patients use the dry powdered devices?
PRELOADED DEVICES
These are quick and simple to use.

The Accuhaler
The Accuhaler device is rotated in its case to expose the mouthpiece and the activating lever is pushed down. The patient takes a deep breath in and breathes out fully, and then places their lips firmly around the mouthpiece and takes a slow steady deep breath in as deeply as possible. The device should be removed from the mouth and the breath held for as long as possible before exhaling slowly. The device is then closed by rotating the case. If further doses are required, the whole process must be repeated.

The Turbohaler
The Turbohaler comes as a short cylinder. The outer case is twisted off. The base is twisted one way until it clicks and then twisted the other way until it can't go any further. The patient then inhales from the device as for the Accuhaler, but it is important that the Turbohaler is held upright – otherwise the primed dose can fall out.

The Twisthaler
The Twisthaler is similar to the Turbohaler. The device is actuated by twisting the cap whilst pressing down.

The Clickhaler
The Clickhaler resembles a stumpy metered-dose aerosol. Pressing the top of the device releases the dose of powdered drug, which can then simply be inhaled through the mouthpiece, in the same way as inhaling through the Accuhaler or Turbohaler. The device must be held vertically once actuated to prevent the powder from falling out.

The Pulvinal
The Pulvinal is a short cylinder with transparent walls, so the patient can see how much dry powder is still available for use. The outer case is unscrewed, and the device is primed by pressing a button on the mouthpiece and twisting the base until a red mark appears in the hole beneath the button. The button is then released and the inhaler twisted in the opposite direction until a green mark appears, with an audible click, below the button. The patient then inhales as for the Turbohaler.

DEVICES THAT REQUIRE LOADING

These are a little more time-consuming and complex to use than preloaded devices.

The Aerohaler

The Aerohaler has six capsules that are loaded into a drum, which is then loaded into the device. A button is pressed to pierce the top and the bottom of the capsule, making the medication available for inhalation.

The Diskhaler

The Diskhaler (Diskus) is available with eight-dose or four-dose discs, depending on the product to be administered. The discs are made from foil and have blisters containing the medication around the edge. The whole disc is inserted into the device. The drug is mixed with the lactose carrier. Once the disc is inserted into the device, the lid of the device is lifted and a spike punctures the disc. The patient then inhales through the mouthpiece, as for the Accuhaler.

The Novolizer

This is available with cartridges containing 100 doses of the drugs to be administered. With the cartridge in the device, the device is 'primed' by pressing the large actuator button. This delivers a metered volume of the dry powder from the cartridge to a cavity underneath the cartridge. Upon inhalation the dry powder is drawn through a turbo device which ensures optimal dispersal of the powder. The counter mechanism counts back after each successful inhalation.

The Spinhaler and the Aerolizer

The actions of the Spinhaler and the Aerolizer devices are very similar. In both devices, the drug is mixed with a lactose-containing powder in a capsule. Each capsule is inserted into the device. The top half of the device is twisted on the bottom half, breaking the capsule and releasing the powder, which can then be inhaled through the mouthpiece.

4.139 What are the advantages and disadvantages of dry powdered devices?

The main advantage of dry powdered inhalers is that they are extremely easy to use. Because the medication leaves the device only when the patient inhales, there are no coordination problems as with metered-dose inhalers. The patient can use several breaths to inhale the dose if necessary. The use of such delivery systems may improve compliance with therapy.

THE ACCUHALER

Advantages: the Accuhaler has a dose counter, enabling drug usage to be monitored and compliance to be checked. It is easy to use and little inspiratory effort is required to obtain the dose. The drug is mixed with lactose to reassure patients that they have taken the dose. It can be used any way up. It is a low resistance device. It is light, portable and its slim shape allows it to fit easily into pockets and handbags. It is available for use with both short-acting and long-acting β_2-agonists, inhaled steroids, and combined steroid and long-acting β_2-agonists.

Disadvantages: It is relatively expensive.

THE TURBOHALER

Advantages: The Turbohaler is easy to use and requires fairly low inspiratory flow rates but, because it is a high-resistance device, more inspirational effort is needed to achieve these flow rates. It probably has the best lung deposition of any device. It has no taste indicator, which is preferred by some patients. It has a display window that shows a red line when only 20 doses are left, or gives an indication of the number of doses left (Symbicort Turbohaler). It is available for use with both short- and long-acting β_2-agonists, inhaled steroids, and combined steroid and long-acting β_2-agonists.

Disadvantages: Its tubular shape is disliked by some, especially if carried in a front trouser pocket. The lack of taste indicator is disliked by some patients as they cannot tell whether they have taken a dose or not. The powder needs to be kept dry because it is not protected from moisture (in the Accuhaler or Diskhaler, the powder is in protective foil blisters), and blowing rather than sucking from the device can lead to dampening of the powder in the Turbohaler and loss of efficacy. It is relatively expensive.

THE CLICKHALER

Advantages: The Clickhaler is easy to use. It is light and compact. It has an integral dose counter, the first panel of which turns red when only ten doses are left. It contains lactose as a taste indicator. Uniquely, it locks when empty, so the patient can be in no doubt as to whether or not they have taken a dose.

Disadvantages: Its shape is a little bulky. It is not available for any long-acting inhaled bronchodilator.

THE PULVINAL

Advantages: The Pulvinal requires low inspiratory flows and has low internal resistance. It allows direct visual assessment of how much powder is left for inhalation. It is relatively inexpensive.

Disadvantages: It is a little more complex to use than other preloaded devices. It is not available for any long-acting inhaled bronchodilator.

THE AEROHALER

Advantages: These are the same as for other dry powdered devices that require preloading.

Disadvantages: The Aerohaler can be used only with ipratroprium. It is relatively expensive.

THE DISKHALER

Advantages: These are as for other dry powdered devices. The shape of the Diskhaler means that it fits easily into pockets and handbags, which makes it quite popular with some patients. It has a taste indicator. It does not require great inspiratory flow. It is available for the complete range of therapies. The blisters are filled precisely during the manufacturing process, helping to ensure accurate and consistent dosing, and the foil protects the medication from moisture.

Disadvantages: The lactose in the powder may make some patients cough. The device may prove a little fiddly for patients to load, especially during acute attacks.

THE NOVOLIZER

Advantages: The Novolizer is easy and quick to use. There is a dose counter which is automatically reset after each dose is taken. If the cartridge is empty, it is impossible to inhale through the device. Very low inspiratory flows are needed to actuate the device.

Disadvantages: It is not available for any long-acting inhaled bronchodilator. It is relatively large and bulky.

THE AEROLIZER AND SPINHALER

Advantages: They are small and easy to use.

Disadvantages: They are quite fiddly, especially during an acute attack. Once loaded, the powder can fall out of the device before inhalation if it is not held correctly. The disadvantage applies, as for Diskhaler and the Turbohaler, if the patient blows rather than sucks. Each device is available for only a single product. The spikes within both devices are quite sharp. They are relatively expensive.

NEBULIZERS

4.140 How do nebulizers work?

Nebulizers work by producing a fine spray of droplets containing the relevant drug. With jet nebulizers, the spray is generated by air or, ideally, oxygen being pumped through a solution containing the appropriate drug and the resultant spray passing to the patient. The spray will still have a forward velocity and therefore requires no inspiratory effort from the patient. A relatively high dose of drug can therefore be given with each nebulization, with no inspiratory effort or coordination required by the patient.

Nebulizers are used for the emergency treatment of acute exacerbations of asthma. They are still used occasionally as regular treatment in infants, especially if they are unable to use a large-volume spacer and mask. In adults, nebulizers are also used for patients unable to obtain control despite correct compliance with full anti-inflammatory therapy and adequate inhaler technique. If used in an emergency, it is preferable to use oxygen to drive the nebulizer.

4.141 What are the advantages and disadvantages of using nebulizers?

ADVANTAGES

Nebulizers deliver a large dose of drug with no effort whatsoever required on behalf of the patient. They are therefore excellent for emergency use. They can be used with short-acting bronchodilators, inhaled steroids (budesonide and fluticasone), ipratropium and cromoglicate.

DISADVANTAGES

Nebulizers are time consuming. They require supervision, and regular cleaning and maintenance. If ipratropium is used in the nebulizer, it is better for the patient to use a mouthpiece rather than a mask in order to minimize the amount of ipratropium being absorbed from the conjunctiva. Nebulizers are also expensive; equipment is bulky and requires a power source.

Patients' overconfidence in their nebulized bronchodilators may lead them to discontinue their preventive therapy or to overuse their bronchodilator therapy. There is concern that patients may rely too heavily on home nebulizers, leading them to delay seeking medical attention and so risk severe life-threatening attacks.

Side-effects may be more marked than with conventional inhalers.

Drugs available for nebulization are very expensive when compared with their equivalents available for use in MDIs plus spacers.

4.142 When should the routine use of nebulizers be recommended?

Regular nebulized bronchodilators should be given only when other methods of drug administration have been tried and rejected, and where there is good compliance with the full range of anti-inflammatory treatments. Increased bronchodilatation without unacceptable effects needs to be shown before this method is continued. A 3 week home trial with peak flow monitoring is advised. Written and verbal instruction should be given to the asthmatic on the method, frequency of use, action to be taken if deterioration occurs, and when to attend for follow-up. Supervision should usually be by a trained asthma nurse or physiotherapist, or at an asthma clinic. Supervision should include prescription monitoring, peak flow evaluation and servicing of the compressor according to the manufacturer's recommendations.

4.143 How should we deal with patients who already have home nebulizers?

In practice, there are many patients whose asthma treatment includes frequent or regular nebulization. Many, if not most, of the patients using nebulizers would find the use of large-volume spacers equally or more effective, but spacers lack the cachet, mystique and allure of the nebulizer. Trying to dissuade patients who have been using nebulizers for months or years that they would be better abandoning the nebulizer for a spacer is difficult – if not impossible. Arguments based on well-conducted research, economics or expert opinions are seldom as persuasive as personal prejudice.

The advantages of weaning patients off nebulizers are many:

■ *Economic*: Nebulized drugs are expensive (especially steroids); nebulizers are expensive to purchase and need at least annual maintenance.
■ *Psychological*: Using 'high-tech' equipment reinforces the sickness role of the patient to themselves and their relatives and friends, and reduces the ability of the patient and their family to regard asthma as a disease that can be controlled rather than one that controls the patient.

Patients and their well-meaning friends and relations should be vigorously dissuaded from buying a nebulizer. Ask them to buy a simple electric fan instead, as many patients with breathing difficulties (from any cause) find symptomatic relief from the effects of cool, moving air.

CHOOSING A DEVICE

4.144 Which devices should we use for children?

In children, particular care must be taken in choosing the delivery system. It is especially important to ensure that a child has sufficient inspiratory flow to get an adequate dose of the drug to the bronchus. Suggested devices for different ages are shown in *Appendix A* [33]

4.145 Which devices should we choose for adults?

Consider:

■ *Patient factors* – Which device does the patient like and which device can they use properly? Many pharmaceutical companies place great store on the inspiratory flows needed in order to inhale fully the dose of medication available from their devices. In practice, most adults and children of school age can manage inspiratory flows well in excess of the minimum needed for each device.

■ *Asthma severity* – Can the patient still reliably use the device even when their asthma is severe? Hopefully this situation will not often occur, but in extreme cases a patient's life may depend on their ability to use the inhaler effectively. If a patient has unstable asthma, or has had severe exacerbations or is at risk of them (especially if long-term compliance may be imperfect), consider a spacer plus MDI for emergency use, or even a nebulizer.

■ *Medication factors* – Not all medications are available in each device. Nearly all medication available as inhaled therapy for asthma comes as MDIs (an exception is formoterol (eformoterol)) and most are available in at least one other device as well.

■ *Economic factors* – MDIs are generally the cheapest devices and, if used properly either alone or via spacers, drug delivery and lung deposition are good; used imperfectly, they are less useful and less cost-effective.

Recommendations:

■ In an adult with full faculties who has an excellent MDI technique, use an MDI, with a spacer if high-dose inhaled steroids are used.

■ For an adult as above but with imperfect MDI technique, use a breath-actuated device (patient to decide which such device he or she prefers; prescriber to ensure technique is adequate).

■ If inhaled long-acting β_2-agonists are needed or likely to be needed, consider the Accuhaler or Turbohaler.

■ If MDI technique is poor and the patient cannot use breath-actuated devices, or does not like them, use a dry powdered device (allow patient to choose which device he or she prefers; prescriber to ensure technique is adequate).

■ For all patients, consider a MDI plus spacer for use if the asthma becomes severe.

■ For all patients, check inhaler technique at least annually, before making any therapeutic changes (increasing or decreasing doses or therapies) and with every exacerbation. Never assume a patient's inhaler technique is adequate. Never assume that a device is so easy to use that the inhaler technique does not need regular checking.

4.146 Which devices should we use for the elderly or disabled?

Patients with visual impairment, tremor, poor coordination (both hand–eye and hand–inspiration) or any combination of these factors are unlikely to be able to use a MDI perfectly, and less likely to be able to use the more complex breath-actuated and dry powdered devices. Consider using:

- Dry powdered devices – the Accuhaler, Clickhaler, Novolizer or Turbohaler
- Breath-actuated devices – the Autohaler or Easibreathe
- A MDI plus spacers.

Avoid use of the Aerohaler, Diskhaler, Pulvinal, Spinhaler and MDIs.

4.147 What about relative costs of asthma therapies?

Bear in mind that the most cost-effective therapies are those that the patient takes correctly and that lead to perfect asthma control and maximum quality of life, and that require minimum input from expensive doctors and nurses. Some drugs cost much more when prescribed in more sophisticated or newer devices. The cheapest therapies are given first:

- Inhaled short-acting β_2-agonists: salbutamol (albuterol) and terbutaline are about the same cost.
- Oral short-acting β_2-agonists: syrup or tablets; salbutamol (albuterol) and terbutaline are about the same cost.
- Inhaled steroids: beclometasone and budesonide are the cheapest; fluticasone is a little more expensive. Higher-dose steroids become more expensive.
- Inhaled anticholinergic agents: higher doses are more expensive, as are the longer-acting agents.
- Oral theophyllines: slow-release preparations are a little more expensive; higher doses become more expensive.
- Oral long-acting β_2-agonists: bambuterol (Bambec) and Volmax are about the same cost, and higher doses cost more.
- Oral leukotriene receptor antagonists: montelukast and zafirleukast cost about the same.
- Inhaled long-acting β_2-agonists: salmeterol and formoterol (eformoterol) are about the same cost.
- Inhaled cromogens: surprisingly expensive.

Appendix B shows the drugs commonly used for asthma, and the devices available for each preparation. *Appendix C* lists the preparations available for each device.

PATIENT QUESTIONS

4.148 Why should I need to take inhaled steroids for my asthma – surely it would be better to avoid whatever causes my asthma?

Trigger avoidance is an option in managing asthma. To be successful, the triggers must be identified and then all exposure to them must be eliminated. Unfortunately, both these tasks are very difficult, if not impossible, for most people with asthma. Nearly all asthmatics have several triggers for their disease, and sometimes a trigger is important only if it occurs when another trigger is also present, such as the combination of having a cold and exercising. There are no guaranteed, completely comprehensive and accurate tests for triggers or allergens. Few people can totally eliminate all their triggers, even if they are all known, and some triggers, such as exercise, are part of normal life and should not be avoided completely; others may give pleasure as well as asthma, such as pets.

The treatments used to control asthma are effective, well tolerated and extremely safe in the usual doses. We also know that if the inflammation in the lungs (which is the root cause of asthma) is controlled with long-term treatment, the person's asthma is likely to remain well controlled and their lungs will be protected from any long-term damage that poorly controlled asthma may cause.

4.149 I find it very difficult to find the time and money I should be spending in trying to reduce the dust and mite exposure in my house. What should I do to help my daughter who has asthma?

Try not to worry too much and don't feel guilty. Anti-house dust mite measures may help some asthmatics some of the time, but they are not vital. It is much more important for you to look after your children in the ways that you are most comfortable with. As long as your child is receiving good asthma care and her asthma is well controlled, and she is able to do all the things she wishes, then you are doing all the right things and providing the best care for your daughter. Just don't smoke in the house (and preferably not at all).

4.150 How can I tell if my asthma is getting better or worse?

If you do not have a self-management or action plan, ask your doctor or nurse for one next time you have an appointment. Otherwise, if you experience any of the following, see your doctor or asthma nurse as soon as you are able:

- Waking at night with coughing, wheezing, shortness of breath or chest tightness
- Increased breathlessness on waking in the morning
- Needing more, or more frequent, relievers, or if you think they aren't working as well or for as long as usual
- If your ability to exercise is worse.

4.151 Are inhaled steroids safe even in children or if used over a long time?

Steroids are natural hormones, made by our bodies, without which we would die. Steroid inhalers or tablets are the best anti-inflammatory drugs available. Asthma is due to inflammation in the lungs. So, it makes sense to use the best available medication to treat asthma. Inhaled steroids are taken in very small doses and are delivered direct to the lungs, so very little of the drug goes into the bloodstream. Therefore, at the doses usually used, inhaled steroids are very safe indeed. There have been literally thousands of studies looking at the long-term effects of taking inhaled steroids, and they have all concluded that inhaled steroids, at the doses usually used, are very safe in the long term. They do not cause any growth suppression.

4.152 Does it matter if I miss the occasional dose of my regular inhalers?

Although little harm will usually occur if you miss the odd dose, it is not advisable. Try to get into the habit of using your preventer puffers twice a day, every day, even when you are well and have been well for a long time. The puffers are designed to keep you well and healthy and to control your asthma, as well as to reduce your risk of an asthma attack.

4.153 If steroids are so safe, why are sportsmen and women not allowed to use them?

Steroid is the name given to a group of hormones that are chemically related. The group includes testosterone and oestrogen as well as the anabolic steroids, which are abused by a few athletes. The steroids used in asthma are called corticosteroids, and they have no effect on body-building or athletic performance; also, the effects of corticosteroids are unrelated to the effects of testosterone and oestrogens.

4.154 How does my doctor or nurse know which treatment is right for me?

He or she will have received training in asthma and its management, and many doctors and nurses have been on postgraduate courses about asthma. They will also be familiar with and use asthma guidelines that have been agreed nationally or internationally. There is a huge amount of research on asthma, and many articles and whole journals are published every week. All the decisions your doctor or nurse makes with you will be based on best available evidence together with the experience of the doctor or nurse, and will take your circumstances and views into account.

4.155 Will treating my asthma help make the disease go away, or will I need to take treatment all my life?

Unfortunately, there is no cure available for asthma at present. Treatment is aimed at controlling the disease, allowing you to lead a normal life and preventing any long-term complications that may occur with poorly managed asthma. Well-managed asthma will usually result in no symptoms and no restrictions, but if the treatment is stopped the disease may well reappear. Some people will need to take preventive treatment all their lives. We know that the outlook for asthma is better in people whose disease is as perfectly controlled as possible for as long as possible.

There are, however, many people whose asthma has remained under good control for many years, and who are then able to taper down their treatment to none and still remain well. Many children seem to fit this pattern.

4.156 Will I get addicted to any of my treatments?

No, none of the treatments used to manage asthma is addictive. Many people worry that the longer they take their treatment for, the more they will need the treatment, or that they will find the treatment less effective over time and need even more. You will not become dependent on the treatment, and neither will you become tolerant to your treatments. You will need to continue taking whatever is needed to control the asthma and enable you to be free of symptoms, but this will not lead to tolerance, dependence or addiction.

Asthma management in practice

ASSESSMENT OF CURRENT MANAGEMENTS

5.1	How well is asthma being managed?	167
5.2	How well is asthma managed in the UK?	167
5.3	Can we make international comparisons on how well asthma is being managed?	168

DEATHS AND ADMISSIONS

| 5.4 | What about hospital admission rates and deaths? | 169 |
| 5.5 | Why have asthma deaths declined in the UK? | 170 |

OUTCOME MEASURES

5,6	What outcome measures are important in asthma?	170
5.7	How can I assess my asthma management of individual patients?	170
5.8	Should I use quality-of-life questionnaires in my practice?	171
5.9	What is the best way to assess my patients?	171
5.10	What are the criteria of good asthma care?	171

TALKING TO PATIENTS

5.11	How do I start with a newly diagnosed asthmatic?	172
5.12	What should I cover at the next few appointments?	172
5.13	What should I cover at subsequent appointments?	172
5.14	Which primary care clinician should manage asthma?	173

PRACTICAL MANAGEMENT

| 5.15 | It all sounds quite easy in theory, but in practice I've got lots of asthmatics whose asthma is difficult to control. Can you advise me on managing different types of difficult asthma? | 174 |

ASTHMA MANAGEMENT: INFANTS (0–2 YEARS)

5.16	How can I diagnose asthma in this age group?	176
5.17	What triggers are relevant when managing asthma in infants?	176
5.18	What medication should I use in infants with asthma?	176

5.19	Should infants have a management plan?	177
5.20	What should I tell parents when I suspect a diagnosis of asthma in their infant?	177
5.21	When should I refer an infant with asthma?	178

ASTHMA MANAGEMENT: TODDLERS AND PRE-SCHOOL-AGED CHILDREN

5.22	How can I diagnose asthma in this age group?	178
5.23	What triggers are relevant when managing asthma in pre-school-aged children?	178
5.24	What medication should I use in pre-school-aged children with asthma?	179
5.25	Should pre-school-aged children have a management plan?	180
5.26	What should I tell parents when I suspect a diagnosis of asthma in their pre-school-aged child?	180
5.27	When should I refer a pre-school-aged child with asthma?	180

ASTHMA MANAGEMENT: SCHOOL-AGED CHILDREN (5–14 YEARS)

5.28	How can I diagnose asthma in this age group?	180
5.29	What triggers are relevant when managing asthma in school-aged children?	180
5.30	What medication should I use in school-aged children with asthma?	181
5.31	How can I help my asthmatic children manage their asthma at school?	181
5.32	How can I help teachers to help my asthmatic patients at school?	182
5.33	Should school-aged children have a management plan?	182
5.34	When should I refer school-aged children with asthma?	182

ASTHMA MANAGEMENT: TEENAGERS WITH ASTHMA

5.35	How can I diagnose asthma in this age group?	182
5.36	What triggers are relevant when managing asthma in teenagers?	183
5.37	What medication should I use for adolescents with asthma?	183
5.38	Should adolescent asthmatics have a management plan?	184
5.39	When should I refer an adolescent with asthma?	184

ASTHMA MANAGEMENT: ADULT ASTHMA

5.40	How can I diagnose asthma in adults?	185
5.41	What triggers are relevant when managing asthma in adults?	185
5.42	What medication should I use for adults with asthma?	185
5.43	Should adult asthmatics have a management plan?	186
5.44	When should I refer an adult with asthma?	186

ASTHMA MANAGEMENT IN PREGNANCY

5.45	What happens to asthma in pregnancy?	186
5.46	What triggers are relevant when managing asthma in pregnancy?	186
5.47	What medication should I use for pregnant women with asthma?	187
5.48	Should pregnant asthmatics have a management plan?	187
5.49	When should I refer a pregnant woman with asthma?	187

MANAGING BRITTLE ASTHMA

5.50	What is brittle asthma and how can I diagnose it?	188
5.51	What triggers are relevant when managing brittle asthma?	188
5.52	What medication should I use in patients with brittle asthma?	188
5.53	Should patients with brittle asthma have a management plan?	189
5.54	When should I refer a patient with brittle asthma?	190

MANAGING MIXED OBSTRUCTIVE AIRWAY DISEASE

5.55	What is mixed obstructive airway disease?	190
5.56	How can I diagnose mixed obstructive airway disease?	190
5.57	What triggers are relevant when managing mixed obstructive airway disease?	191
5.58	What medication should I use in mixed obstructive airway disease?	191
5.59	Should patients with mixed obstructive airway disease have a management plan?	192
5.60	When should I refer patients with mixed obstructive airways disease, or should I manage them in my asthma clinic?	192

MANAGING OCCUPATIONAL ASTHMA

5.61	What is meant by occupational asthma?	193
5.62	How common is it?	193

5.63	What are the most common causes of occupational asthma?	193
5.64	How can I diagnose occupational asthma?	194
5.65	How should I manage occupational asthma?	194
5.66	What about a career in the armed forces for asthmatic patients?	195

MANAGING ASTHMA IN THE ELDERLY

5.67	How can I diagnose asthma in this age group?	195
5.68	What triggers are relevant when managing asthma in the elderly?	196
5.69	What medication should I use in elderly patients with asthma?	196
5.70	Should elderly asthmatics have a management plan?	196
5.71	When should I refer elderly patients with asthma?	196

MANAGING DIFFICULT ASTHMA

| 5.72 | A few of my patients seem to have troublesome symptoms and sudden changes in asthma control despite small falls in their peak flow readings. Why is this and how should I manage them? | 197 |
| 5.73 | I also have a few patients who don't seem to appreciate that their asthma has become very severe until quite late. How can I help them? | 197 |

COMPLIANCE

5.74	One of the biggest problems I have is getting my patients to comply with the suggested management. Why is this and how can I improve compliance?	198
5.75	Is poor compliance just due to patients' ignorance?	198
5.76	Are there different types of non-compliance?	198
5.77	How can I improve my patients' compliance?	199
5.78	How can I get my patients to take their inhaled steroids?	199

SMOKING AND ASTHMA

| 5.79 | Is smoking a problem in asthma? | 200 |
| 5.80 | How can I help my patients stop smoking? | 201 |

MANAGING ASTHMA IN PATIENTS WITH OTHER DISEASES

| 5.81 | Many of my asthma patients have other disorders. Will their asthma management be different? | 201 |

EXERCISE-INDUCED ASTHMA

| 5.82 | What is exercise-induced asthma? | 202 |

5.83 How can I diagnose exercise-induced asthma? 202

5.84 How should I manage exercise-induced asthma? 203

5.85 What medications are useful in exercise-induced asthma? 203

5.86 What about longer-term management and prevention of exercise-induced asthma? 204

5.87 What about professional or representative sports – are there any problems with taking asthma medications? 204

5.88 Surely asthma must be a handicap at some levels of sport? 205

MANAGING TROUBLESOME SYMPTOMS

5.89 What is cough variant asthma? 205

5.90 What should I do if the asthma seems to be persistently worse at night? 206

5.91 What is the role of respiratory infections? Many of my asthmatic patients seem to get chest infections. 206

5.92 Should all my asthmatic patients avoid aspirin? 207

5.93 Some of my female asthmatic patients say that the severity of their asthma alters with their menstrual cycle. How can I help them? 207

ASTHMA AND TRAVEL

5.94 What advice should I give to asthmatics about travelling? 208

5.95 What advice should I give to asthmatics about flying? 208

PRIMARY PREVENTION OF ASTHMA

5.96 Can asthma be prevented? 209

5.97 What advice can we give to a prospective mother worried that her children may develop asthma? 210

5.98 Can environmental changes reduce the risks of developing asthma? 210

REFRACTIVE ASTHMA

5.99 What do I do with the asthmatic who is not getting better despite all my efforts? 211

5.100 What can I do about patients who frequently attend the local accident and emergency department or walk-in centre? 213

5.101 Why and when should I follow-up patients who have been seen in the hospital or walk-in centre? 213

GUIDELINES AND PROTOCOLS

5.102	When were asthma guidelines introduced in the UK?	214
5.103	Why do we need the latest BTS/SIGN guidelines?	214
5.104	What is new in the 2002 BTS/SIGN asthma guidelines?	215
5.105	Why do some organizations have their own guidelines as well?	215
5.106	What is the difference between a guideline and a protocol?	215
5.107	What should a practice protocol for asthma contain?	216
5.108	How often should we review well patients?	216
5.109	Who should review the patients?	216
5.110	What should we do at the review appointment?	217

AUDIT

5.111	What is audit?	217
5.112	Why audit asthma care?	217
5.113	What are the principles behind auditing my asthma care?	217
5.114	What do I need to audit?	218
5.115	What do I do with my audit results?	218
5.116	What should I audit?	218
5.117	How do I collect the data?	219
5.118	What do I do with these data?	220
5.119	How do I know what changes to make?	220
5.120	How do I make the necessary changes?	220
5.121	Isn't audit a bit boring and depressing?	221
5.122	Does audit show that asthma clinics make any difference to the provision of asthma care?	221
5.123	What about more sophisticated audits?	221

ASSESSMENT OF CURRENT MANAGEMENTS

5.1 How well is asthma being managed?

Compared with the management of asthma 20 years ago, the answer is very well, but compared with the standards laid down by national and international guidelines, there is still room for a great deal of improvement.

The Asthma Insights and Reality in Europe (AIRE) study[1] surveyed nearly 300 asthmatics throughout Europe and found that the Global Initiatives for Asthma (GINA) standards were not being met:

■ More than half or all adult respondents and a third of all children reported daytime symptoms at least once a week.

■ More than half of all adults and children reported asthma episodes in the previous month.

■ Most adults and children had needed to use their relievers in the previous month.

■ More than half of the children and nearly half of the adults claimed that they had never had any lung function tests.

Studies from the USA[2] and the International Study of Asthma and Allergies in Childhood (ISAAC) study[3] confirm that asthma morbidity is still high, even in countries with sophisticated healthcare systems. Overall, more than a quarter of children with current asthma reported more than four attacks within the previous year. The European Community Respiratory Health Survey[4] found that one in three adults with current asthma had had nocturnal breathlessness in the previous year.

5.2 How well is asthma managed in the UK?

In the UK there have been many large surveys on the effects of asthma:

■ In the 1990–1 National Asthma Survey[5] involving 61 000 respondents, Action Asthma found that nearly half of the respondents experienced symptoms on most days. Most asthmatics were woken at least once a week by their symptoms. One in five respondents thought that asthma had a major effect on their lives, but many were so used to their restrictive lifestyle that they no longer regarded these restrictions as abnormal.

■ In 1993 Action Asthma conducted a similar survey amongst asthmatic children. The Young Asthmatics Survey[6] received over 20 000 responses from children aged 4–17 years in the UK. As with the adult survey, the results showed that many asthmatic children were inadequately controlled, resulting in a compromised lifestyle. One in three children were woken at least once a week by the asthma, and nearly a quarter had symptoms on most days.

■ In the National Asthma Campaign's Impact of Asthma Survey,[7] asthmatic respondents were recruited by leaflets that were left in doctors' surgeries, supermarkets, community centres and pharmacies. The survey was carried out in the autumn of 1995, and 44 000 responses were analysed. Some 25% of respondents felt that asthma controlled their life or had a major effect on it, and 40% experienced asthma symptoms on most days. A similar number were woken at night at least once a week with asthma symptoms.

■ The 2002 Asthma Control and Expectations Survey[8] showed that many asthmatics alter their lifestyle to avoid asthma symptoms. More than half of respondents accepted a restricted lifestyle as the price to be paid for feeling well.

5.3 Can we make international comparisons on how well asthma is being managed?

This is always difficult because the data may not be collected in the same way in different countries, and definitions of, for example, acute asthma may vary. The mortality rates for asthma have actually increased in the USA. This may be due to the lower use of inhaled steroids in the United States, and the subsequent failure of disease modification and suppression of airway inflammation, although other factors such as access to health care

TABLE 5.1 Comparison of asthma statistics in various countries

Country	Asthma mortality rate per 100 000 (1993)	Prevalence of severe asthma (1993–5) (%)	Ratio
Australia	0.86	8.3	0.10
Canada	0.25	8.1	0.03
England	0.52	8.5	0.06
Finland	0.21	3.1	0.07
France	0.40	2.8	0.14
Germany	0.44	5.7	0.08
Italy	0.23	2.0	0.12
Japan	0.73	2.1	0.35
New Zealand	0.50	8.0	0.06
Sweden	0.12	2.0	0.06
USA	0.47	10.0	0.05

From Beasley and Mazoli[9] by kind permission of the editor

and medication are also important. Death rates are higher in disadvantaged, poorly educated and urban populations.

A useful measure when comparing outcomes of asthma care between countries is the ratio of the asthma mortality rate to the prevalence rate of severe asthma in each country. Bear in mind that there are difficulties in standardizing descriptions of severe asthma, and of obtaining age-matched data. The lower the ratio, the 'better' the asthma outcomes, as shown in *Table 5.1*.[9]

DEATH AND ADMISSIONS

5.4   What about hospital admission rates and deaths?

These rates have increased dramatically in the UK over the past 20 years, but are beginning to decline again from a peak in the early 1990s; the decline is for all age groups, but is especially marked for children and young adults, as shown in *Table 5.2*.[10] *Table 5.3* shows the trends in hospital admission rates for different age groups between 1979 and 1999 in England and Wales.[10]

TABLE 5.2 Percentage change from 1979 to 1999 in admission and mortality rates for asthma in England and Wales

Age band (years)	HOSPITAL ADMISSIONS		MORTALITY	
	1999 rate (per 10 000)	Change from 1979 to 1999 (%)	1999 rate (per 10^6)	Change from 1979 to 1999 (%)
0–4	58.3	+118	1.8	–40
5–14	18.2	+29	2.4	–37
15–44	9.0	+73	6.2	–43
45–64	8.9	+27	23.6	–38
65+	9.8	+49	110.2	+3

TABLE 5.3 Trends in hospital admission rates for asthma in adults and children, England and Wales 1979–99

Age band (years)	Admission rate per 10 000 population							
	1979	1982	1985	1988	1991	1994	1997	1999
Children								
0–4	23	44	81	101	98	83	74	64
5–15	18	21	24	26	25	24	19	19
Adults								
15–44	5	6	8	10	10	10	9	9
45–64	7	9	12	11	10	10	9	9
65+	7	9	10	10	10	11	9	9

Also, the mortality rate in the UK has declined against a background of rising prevalence of asthma, so that the rate per 1000 diagnosed asthmatics has reduced substantially, especially in adults. *See also Q. 3.10.*

5.5   Why have asthma deaths declined in the UK?

The reduction in asthma deaths is widely considered to be due to improved asthma management, especially the more widespread use of inhaled steroids.

OUTCOME MEASURES

5.6   What outcome measures are important in asthma?

Clinicians and patients should aim for perfection in managing asthma. The overall aim should be to maintain perfect control of the disease and prevent any future problems. More specifically:

- No or minimal symptoms during the day and at night
- Normal or best-possible lung function – peak expiratory flow (PEF) or forced expiratory volume in 1 second (FEV_1)
- Unimpeded, appropriate lifestyle with ability to exercise and work as easily as one's peers
- No or minimal need for medical input, especially urgently – this implies no acute episodes of asthma
- Minimal use and need for relieving medication
- Management, including medication, that is safe and minimally disruptive.

The mission statement of the Swindon Asthma Group states these aims succinctly:

> 'Every asthmatic should lead a normal life untroubled by their disease or its management.'

5.7   How can I assess my asthma management of individual patients?

The list of outcome measures is too long and vague to be a series of questions to patients. The Royal College of General Physicians[11] has formulated three questions as a means of rapidly assessing an asthmatic patient's control:

- Have you had any difficulty in sleeping because of your asthma or cough in the last week?
- Have you had any of your usual asthma symptoms (cough, wheeze, chest tightness or shortness of breath) in the last week?

■ Has your asthma interfered with your your usual activities (work, school, exercise, chores) in the last month?

Although useful, these questions have not been fully validated and provide no information on the effect of these symptoms on the patient's overall well-being. It is the way in which a patient reacts and adapts to symptoms, rather than the symptoms themselves, that determine how having a chronic disease affects an individual.

5.8 Should I use quality-of-life questionnaires in my practice?

Various quality-of-life questionnaires are used in research projects, but their use for individual patients is time consuming. The information that these questionnaires give is not specific enough to allow evaluation of changes in management, but provides an overall assessment of well-being, so they are not often used in clinical practice.

5.9 What is the best way to assess my patients?

There is no formula or short cut that will be applicable to every patient. We are left with taking a personal history for each patient. We should try to include symptoms, loss of function, and reaction to the symptoms and management, concentrating on the factors that are most important to the patient.

5.10 What are the criteria of good asthma care?

The patient:
■ Is aware of their diagnosis
■ Is aware of what asthma is, and the principles of its management
■ Has continuing involvement in their asthma management, especially with regard to choice of inhaler device
■ Has minimal symptoms
■ Can sleep through the night
■ Can do whatever exercise and work is appropriate
■ Needs their relieving inhaler rarely or not at all
■ Can lead a normal lifestyle minimally troubled by either the asthma or its management
■ Has managed to eliminate or reduce any triggers with minimal or no disruption to their preferred lifestyle
■ Knows exactly how and when to recognize when their asthma is deteriorating, how and when to alter their own treatment, and how and when to call for help
■ Has their lung function monitored regularly (if appropriate and possible) and the FEV_1 shows no excess decline with age.

TALKING TO PATIENTS

5.11 How do I start with a newly diagnosed asthmatic?

At the initial appointment:

- Register the patient
- Measure height and weight
- Explain the purpose of the clinic (it is not just for ill asthmatics)
- Complete the summary or database card or computer screen including past history, family history, current and past medications for asthma, allergies
- Teach and check inhaler technique
- Teach and check peak flow reading if appropriate
- Assess the severity of asthma from the recent history, drug use and lifestyle
- Identify triggers
- Arrange a subsequent appointment for 1–2 weeks' time.

5.12 What should I cover at the next few appointments?

- Explore the patient's assessment of their disease.
- Explain about the disease and its management.
- Ask about symptom control. Be as specific as possible. Ask especially about days off work or school, night symptoms, exercise tolerance, and any limitations of daily living. Ask about the patient's partner's sleep disturbance by the patient's symptoms.
- Ask whether the patient can do all the things they would like to do.
- Ask them how often they need to use their reliever inhaler.
- Review the trigger factors and, if possible, their avoidance.
- Check peak flow readings if appropriate.
- Explain the concept of peak flow readings and prescribe a peak flow meter if appropriate.
- Make sure the patient knows how to recognize deterioration, how to respond, and how to call for help.
- Check the inhaler technique and adjust if necessary.
- Check compliance.
- Listen to the patient.
- Explain and educate if necessary.
- Arrange a follow-up appointment.

5.13 What should I cover at subsequent appointments?

Subsequent appointments should cover:

- Symptom control
- Inhaler technique

- Compliance with drugs
- Patient's confidence about when to increase treatment, how to do it, and when to call for help
- Answer any questions
- Enquire about how asthma and its management may be affecting the lifestyle of the asthmatic.

5.14 Which primary care clinician should manage asthma?

General practice in the UK is able to provide comprehensive personal, family and community care that includes chronic disease management, as the primary healthcare team provides a wide range of care.

THE PRACTICE NURSE

Properly supported and trained practice nurses can manage the majority of patients with asthma in primary care; in the UK the bulk of this care is provided by the nurses. To be effective, nurses do need ongoing training and updating, and the support of their general practitioner and managerial colleagues.

THE COMMUNITY OR DISTRICT NURSE

Community nurses can be aware of potential asthmatics in the community who may not have been diagnosed. They can also be aware of 'neglected' asthmatics who have not been reviewed or seen for their asthma for some time. They are in a unique position for assessing many housebound patients who are known to be asthmatic or who might have asthma. Alternatively, some community nurses may be able to assess the patients themselves, especially if the nurse has been properly trained and supported; such nurses can fulfil the same role as the practice nurse in the asthma clinic, but working in the patient's own home.

THE HEALTH VISITOR

Health visitors regularly see new babies and their mothers, as well as providing ongoing care and assessment of, especially, the under-fives in either their own home or health visitor clinics. They are therefore in a good position to advise mothers of young children on the management of any child's asthma, and on primary and secondary prevention.

THE COMMUNITY MIDWIFE

Like the health visitor, the community midwife is in an excellent position to provide ongoing care, advice and education to known asthmatic mothers or mothers-to-be.

THE SCHOOL NURSE

The school nurse can provide ongoing support and education to any known asthmatics at the school. She can also advise and educate teachers on asthma and its treatment, so that children who are having symptoms at school can be properly and adequately treated with minimal disruption to either the child or the rest of the class.

THE PAEDIATRIC LIAISON NURSE

This type of nurse is employed by some Trusts or health authorities to liaise between the hospital paediatric department and primary care. Her role is one of facilitating seamless care between primary and secondary providers. She can provide ongoing support and education for patients and their families. She can also check on inhaler technique and compliance.

PHYSIOTHERAPISTS

Physiotherapists in the community can help with the education, compliance and inhaler technique of known asthmatics.

PHARMACISTS

Pharmacists can have a role in the care of asthma, both by supplying medicines and by advising and motivating patients. Pharmacists also have a role in advising asthmatic patients on the unsuitability of treating their symptoms with proprietary cough and cold mixtures. They can encourage patients to seek professional medical help if their symptoms are deteriorating.

PRACTICAL MANAGEMENT

5.15 It all sounds quite easy in theory, but in practice I've got lots of asthmatics whose asthma is difficult to control. Can you advise me on managing different types of difficult asthma?

Asthma management is logical and usually straightforward, but we all have patients who have asthma that is difficult to control. It is probably easier to consider the components of managing asthma, and then to apply these components to various categories and types of patient.

There are five major steps in managing asthma in primary care.

1 The diagnosis

- The diagnosis must be suspected and proven.
- The diagnosis must be agreed and accepted by the members of the primary healthcare team, the patient and the patient's carers (if appropriate).

■ Other possible diagnoses should also be considered in each case, and steps taken to differentiate the diagnosis as accurately as possible.

2 Triggers

■ For each asthmatic, the triggers for their asthma must be identified if possible.

■ Avoidance of any likely triggers should be discussed and, if feasible and agreed to be worthwhile by both the patient and the doctor or nurse, appropriate avoidance measures should be agreed and undertaken.

3 Drug treatment

■ Particular attention must be placed on each patient using the most appropriate *device* that they are happy and able to use. Ideally each patient should be able to take all his or her medication by using one form of device, although sometimes a different device may be needed for use away from home.

■ No drug is effective unless taken correctly and so the correct *technique* of using the device should be checked regularly.

■ Some patients may need to change their devices, depending on their changing circumstances. For example, a device that was suitable for a small infant may be less suitable once the child starts school.

4 Self-management plans

■ Each patient should be capable of monitoring the severity of their own asthma, either by recognizing changes in their symptoms or by additionally using peak flow measurements. The patient must then be capable of knowing how and when to increase treatment, and how and when to call for help.

■ These self-management plans can be successful only if there is good education of the patients by members of the primary healthcare team regarding asthma and its management. Other essential platforms of successful asthma management are good compliance with the treatment regimens and good inhaler technique.

5 Sharing

■ Management of asthma is dependent on agreement between a patient and their carers within the primary healthcare team. Often, further sharing of management will be needed with secondary care. The patient will also need to share their management with their immediate family, and often with their school or workplace.

These five bases provide the framework for the successful management of asthma. More specific details of particular problems that may be encountered in primary care when managing asthma will now be discussed, using the five bases as a common framework.

> Most problems in managing asthma are due to poor education, poor sharing of knowledge, skills and attitudes, and subsequent undertreatment. Asthma continues frequently to be undertreated, suggesting continual opportunities to reduce its morbidity by the more consistent application of existing guidelines.

ASTHMA MANAGEMENT: INFANTS (0–2 YEARS)

5.16 How can I diagnose asthma in this age group?

The diagnosis is usually based on recurrent coughing, especially at night, either in the absence of upper respiratory tract infection, or that is disproportionate to the severity of the infection, or cough that persists for more than a few days beyond the coryzal episode. The younger the child, the more difficult it is to make the diagnosis. A positive response to bronchodilator treatment will strongly support the diagnosis, especially if the success is repeated. Be more suspicious if the child has a strong family history of atopy. Be wary of infants who may have asthma-like symptoms but who were born prematurely, or were intubated, especially if they were also ventilated and spent time in a special care baby unit after birth. It is probable that such children are more at risk of developing asthma in later infancy, but they may also have upper airway stenosis or bronchopulmonary dysplasia. Be mindful also that the child may have croup, bronchiolitis or whooping cough, the latter being more likely in unvaccinated children. Some infants may have acid reflux that presents purely as a cough, which may be worse at night. A rarer but important differential diagnosis is cystic fibrosis. The sudden onset of symptoms should make one suspect an inhaled foreign body. *See also Q. 2.3 and Q. 2.29*

5.17 What triggers are relevant when managing asthma in infants?

The most common trigger is upper respiratory tract infection. The role of the house dust mite is probably also very important. On no account should the family pet be allowed into the child's bedroom at any time. No child at any age should be exposed to cigarette smoking, and the parents should be strongly encouraged to stop smoking and to realize that it is not acceptable just to agree to smoking 'not in front of the baby'.

5.18 What medication should I use in infants with asthma?
BRONCHODILATORS

Inhaled short-acting β_2-agonists as needed are the first-line therapy. Response to bronchodilators may be very variable. There is little evidence that anticholinergic drugs are superior bronchodilators in infants.

INHALED STEROIDS

Long-term anti-inflammatory treatment with inhaled corticosteroids may not always be needed, and it is still not certain that inhaled corticosteroids alter the natural history of asthma in this age group. While there is increasing evidence that inhaled steroids should be started and maintained in the long term – as soon after diagnosis as possible in established asthma – there is still some concern about the effects of long-term inhaled steroids on the development of the lungs in very small infants, especially in the first six months of life. Referral for a second opinion from a paediatrician with an interest in asthma may be advisable before committing small infants to long-term inhaled steroids. The younger the child, the greater the need for a second opinion.

DEVICES

To deliver inhaled therapy, small infants require a large-volume spacer plus face mask, held vertically so as to allow the valve to open and remain open. If the parents and infant cannot manage the spacers, a nebulizer can be tried. Be aware that paroxysmal bronchoconstriction can occasionally occur with nebulized bronchodilators.

5.19 Should infants have a management plan?

The type and duration of treatment needed in infants will depend entirely on each infant's response to the treatments. There are no objective assessments of airway obstruction in small infants that can easily be used by parents or general practitioners. In general, most infants can be managed by using short courses of inhaled short-acting bronchodilators on an as-required basis using a large-volume spacer, but parents and carers will need to know how to recognize deterioration (usually increased cough, especially at night, reluctance to feed, rapid respiration and fretfulness) and to seek help if they suspect any deterioration.

5.20 What should I tell parents when I suspect a diagnosis of asthma in their infant?

All parents naturally want their children to be perfectly healthy and may resist a diagnosis of a chronic, incurable disorder. However, many parents may already have considered the diagnosis themselves, and many will be relieved that there is an explanation for their child's symptoms and that they have a treatable condition. When considering the diagnosis of asthma in this age group, share the uncertainty with the parents and explain the difficulties of making a firm diagnosis. Explain to them that response to treatment is one of the pillars of diagnosis and that is why it is best to treat before a firm diagnosis is made (indeed it is often inevitable). Explanation and education about asthma is always important, particularly for parents of very young children. Frequent reviews of the baby and parents will be necessary, especially initially.

5.21 When should I refer an infant with asthma?

- Be especially ready to refer babies to a paediatrician if there is any doubt about the diagnosis or management.
- Refer all babies under the age of 6 months for assessment, and also any child who has spent time in a special care baby unit, especially if the baby was ventilated or premature.
- Refer before starting an infant on long-term inhaled steroids. Unless you are quite experienced and confident, giving a course of oral steroids to young babies as a diagnostic test is probably best left to specialists.
- Be prepared to discuss the baby's asthma and its management, with parental permission, with crèche workers, nannies or childminders, if appropriate.

ASTHMA MANAGEMENT: TODDLERS AND PRE-SCHOOL-AGED CHILDREN

5.22 How can I diagnose asthma in this age group?

The main symptoms in children of this age are coughing, especially at night, or symptoms with or following a cold that persist for more than a few days after the cold has finished. Children are generally well otherwise and do not have failure to thrive or gastrointestinal symptoms. Peak flow readings are not sufficiently reliable in this age group.

The main differential diagnoses in this age group are simple cough with upper respiratory tract infection, croup, bronchiolitis, whooping cough (especially in the unvaccinated) and persistent postnasal drip. Other possible diagnoses include recurrent gastro-oesophageal reflux with aspiration and chronic upper respiratory tract infections. A rarer but important differential diagnosis is cystic fibrosis. The sudden onset of symptoms should make one suspect an inhaled foreign body. *See Q. 2.29*

5.23 What triggers are relevant when managing asthma in pre-school-aged children?

Identification of likely triggers is usually obtained by taking a careful history. Colds, upper respiratory tract infections and exercise are the commonest triggers. Many asthmatic children have atopy; many are allergic to the house dust mite and a smaller number to animal dander. It is reasonable to give all children and their parents some basic advice on reducing exposure to house dust mite and animal dander by, for instance, not allowing pets into the bedroom at any time, and giving general advice about buying new mattresses and damp-dusting bedrooms. More intensive anti-house dust mite avoidance is more expensive and time consuming, and needs individual assessment with regard to the benefits and costs. General advice about avoiding pollens if the asthma is seasonal is usually fairly straightforward. Skin prick tests can be used in children but are seldom available in the UK, and the tests are not as important as a close and careful history. The results of skin prick tests may sometimes be misleading and may not help with clinical management at all. No child should ever be exposed to cigarette smoke (*see Q. 2.20*).

5.24 What medication should I use in pre-school-aged children with asthma?

All pre-school children with asthma require a short-acting bronchodilator. Most need regular inhaled steroids for control and the prevention of future problems. A small number require third-line agents:

- Leukotriene receptor antagonsists (LTRAs), especially if exercise seems to be a major trigger
- Inhaled long-acting β_2-agonists (licensed only for children aged 4 years or more)
- Oral theophyllines, usually slow-release and low-to-medium dose (beware side-effects, which are common)
- High-dose inhaled steroids
- Oral long-acting bronchodilators.

The best inhaler devices for pre-school-aged children are the large-volume spacers. Smaller children need the mask attachment, and the spacer should be held vertically to keep the valve open. As children grow older, they can discard the mask. Devices for children are shown in *Table 5.4*.

TABLE 5.4 Device selection for children	
Age (years)	**Inhalation delivery system**
< 2	Large-volume spacer plus mask with metered-dose inhaler
	Nebulizer
2–4	Large-volume spacer with metered-dose inhaler
	Nebulizer for emergencies
4–8	Dry powder devices
	Large-volume spacer with inhaler for emergencies
> 8	Dry powder devices
	Metered-dose inhaler
	Breath-actuated inhaler

5.25 Should pre-school-aged children have a management plan?

Some children of pre-school age who have asthma can be well maintained by using short-acting bronchodilators intermittently, with more regular use in response to upper respiratory tract infections. Most children will need long-term preventive treatment as well. Parents should know when to increase the treatment, usually in response to an increase in symptoms or to a cold or other upper respiratory tract infection.

5.26 What should I tell parents when I suspect a diagnosis of asthma in their pre-school-aged child?

Often the diagnosis is received with some relief by parents, who may have felt for some time that something was amiss with their child. Share the diagnosis and emphasize that there are safe and effective treatments for asthma (rather than the multiple courses of antibiotics that the child may have been given in the past).

5.27 When should I refer a pre-school-aged child with asthma?

Referral to a paediatrician is again advisable if:

- There is diagnostic uncertainty
- The asthma is proving difficult to control
- Before contemplating long-term high-dose inhaled steroids
- There is significant co-morbidity (such as heart disease, cystic fibrosis, metabolic disorder).

ASTHMA MANAGEMENT: SCHOOL-AGED CHILDREN (5–14 YEARS)

5.28 How can I diagnose asthma in this age group?

As children get older, the diagnosis becomes more straightforward. Many children present with episodic wheeze, cough, breathlessness and chest tightness (children often complain that their chest hurts or aches), especially on exertion and at night.

The differential diagnosis includes recurrent gastro-oesophageal reflux with aspiration and chronic upper respiratory tract infections. Acute bronchitis may occasionally occur. Even children at primary school can inhale foreign bodies.

5.29 What triggers are relevant when managing asthma in school-aged children?

- By the time children go to school, the identification of likely triggers from taking a careful history is usually more straightforward.

■ As with all children, avoidance of tobacco smoke is imperative.
■ Pets should not be allowed into the bedrooms.
■ General methods to reduce house dust mites are probably reasonable to suggest, especially if the child is atopic.
■ Skin prick testing can be used with the same proviso as discussed above (*see Q. 2.20 and Q. 5.23*).

5.30 What medication should I use in school-aged children with asthma?

BRONCHODILATORS

All children should have ready access to inhaled short-acting β_2-agonists. Most children will require regular, long-term inhaled steroids (<400 μg/day). A smaller number will also require one or more of the following (in order):

1 Inhaled long-acting β_2-agonists.
2 Oral LTRAs, especially if exercise is a major trigger. If compliance with inhaled therapy is irredeemable, LTRAs can be used as sole therapy. This strategy is commonly used in the USA but European clinicians are less keen, and are wary of denying children the long-term benefits of inhaled steroids.
3 Oral theophyllines (beware side-effects; use low to medium doses).
4 High-dose inhaled steroids (400–800 μg/day).
5 Oral long-acting β_2-agonists.

DEVICES

Although metered-dose inhalers (MDIs) with large-volume spacers are the cheapest and most effective option, children naturally find them too bulky to carry to school. They could use them for their twice-daily medication at home, with a second device for their as-needed bronchodilator, but most children will prefer to use all their medications using the same type of inhaler device. Choose the device with the child, and be aware of which devices currently and locally carry the most prestige. Most dry-powder devices are suitable and many children can use breath-actuated MDIs. Even children as young as 5 years can safely be left in charge of their own inhalers, as long as they are suitably instructed. Devices for children are shown in *Table 5.4.*

5.31 How can I help my asthmatic children manage their asthma at school?

Many children's asthma will be well controlled by regular inhaled steroids taken at home, and they will not have any symptoms in school. However, a significant number will have problems, especially with exercise, and may need relieving treatments. Children should, unless there are compelling reasons against, always have access to their own relieving inhalers and be allowed to use them when they feel the need. Children and parents will need guidance on this from their doctor or nurse.

5.32 How can I help teachers to help my asthmatic patients at school?

■ Liaison with the teachers and school nurse may be desirable or necessary, and an agreed policy on allowing asthmatics access to their own medication may be needed.

■ Teachers at school should have access to a large-volume spacer with a metered-dose short-acting bronchodilator that can be used for any child who is having acute symptoms. A protocol may need to be agreed by the school or education authority and the local health authority or community health services, involving local primary healthcare teams and school nurses as well as teachers.

■ Teachers will need teaching so they find asthma less confusing and frightening, and they are able to offer their asthmatic pupils the most appropriate help and support.

■ Asthmatic children should be encouraged to join in all activities and sports, and must not be stigmatized or discriminated against.

5.33 Should school-aged children have a management plan?

By the time a child attends primary school, he or she should be involved with the education about their disease and should be an active participant in discussing its management. As children grow older, they should take increasing responsibility for managing their asthma and for their own compliance.

Simple plans should be agreed verbally, more complex ones written down. Examples of plans are shown in *Figs 4.2 and 4.3*.

5.34 When should I refer school-aged children with asthma?

Referral to a paediatrician is again advisable:

■ If there is diagnostic uncertainty
■ If the asthma is proving difficult to control
■ Before contemplating long-term high-dose inhaled steroids
■ If there is significant co-morbidity (such as heart disease, cystic fibrosis, metabolic disorder).

ASTHMA MANAGEMENT: TEENAGERS WITH ASTHMA

5.35 How can I diagnose asthma in this age group?

Asthma is the most common chronic disease of adolescence. Most teenagers with asthma have the condition diagnosed as primary school or pre-school children. However, asthma can begin at any age and the teenage years are no exception. Often, asthma first presents with exercise-induced symptoms, and it is during the teenage years that many children begin to exercise more competitively or vigorously. Older teenagers will present with coughing, wheeze, shortness of breath and chest tightness, just like adult asthmatics.

Many teenagers are reluctant to accept a new diagnosis of asthma or that their continuing respiratory symptoms are due to continuing childhood asthma, especially if they have been erroneously promised that they will 'grow out of it'.

The main differential diagnoses are postnasal drip or persistent upper respiratory tract infection, including chronic sinusitis.

5.36 What triggers are relevant when managing asthma in teenagers?

- Trigger identification and avoidance are similar to measures advised for younger children.
- Actively discourage smoking.
- Avoidance of passive smoking in the home is also advisable, but it can be more difficult for adolescents to avoid passive smoking in pubs, clubs or discos.
- Anecdotal advice that illicit drugs such as marijuana can benefit asthma should never be condoned as part of the conventional treatment of asthma. Most marijuana is taken mixed with tobacco, so is bound to be damaging to the lungs.
- Many teenagers will begin working either as part of their work experience or after leaving school, and will be exposed to new triggers and allergens in the workplace. Again, a careful history is required in each case to help identify any work-related asthma. Management of occupational asthma is discussed more fully in Q. 5.65.

5.37 What medication should I use for adolescents with asthma?

BRONCHODILATORS

All patients should have ready access to inhaled short-acting β_2-agonists. Most will require regular long-term use of inhaled steroids (<400 µg/day rising to 800 µg/day in older adolescents). A smaller number will also require one or more of the following (in order):

1　Inhaled long-acting β_2-agonists.
2　Oral LTRAs, especially if exercise is a major trigger. If compliance with inhaled therapy is irredeemable, LTRAs can be used as sole therapy. This strategy is commonly used in the USA, but European clinicians are less keen, and are wary of denying children the long-term benefits of inhaled steroids.

3 Oral theophyllines (beware side-effects; use low to medium doses).
4 High-dose inhaled steroids (800–2000 µg/day in older adolescents).
5 Oral long-acting β_2-agonists.

DEVICES

Any of the inhaler devices is suitable, as long as the patient can use it correctly. Choose with the patient, taking into account which devices are currently trendy, but also the shape and size of the device and how easy it is to use unobtrusively.

5.38 Should adolescent asthmatics have a management plan?

Yes:

■ Good control avoids the embarrassment of symptoms or having to use treatments in public. Adolescence is a difficult enough time for most of us, without any additional burden from a chronic disease or its management.

■ It is especially important to involve all adolescents in managing their own disorder.

■ Do not assume that all adolescents are hostile to their diagnosis or its management, or that they will deny they have asthma, but be aware that these are always possibilities.

■ Be aware that poorly controlled asthma in this age group may *not* be simply the result of adolescent rebellion and poor compliance.

■ Simple plans should be agreed verbally, more complex ones written down. Examples of plans are shown in *Figs 4.2 and 4.3*.

■ The responsibility for asthma management needs to be transferred during adolescence from the family to the individual. We can help facilitate this transfer by treating the adolescent appropriately: partly as an adult when needed and partly as a child when needed.

5.39 When should I refer an adolescent with asthma?

Referral to a paediatrician or adult physician is advisable if:

■ There is diagnostic uncertainty
■ The asthma is proving difficult to control
■ Before contemplating long-term high-dose inhaled steroids
■ There is significant co-morbidity (such as heart disease, cystic fibrosis, metabolic disorder).

Some hospitals have special clinics for adolescent asthmatics; others may have 'change-over' clinics where older children requiring long-term follow-up can be transferred to an adult physician by the paediatrician.

ASTHMA MANAGEMENT: ADULT ASTHMA

5.40   How can I diagnose asthma in adults?

Many children with asthma lose their asthmatic tendency as they get older, and many will be completely asymptomatic by the time they reach early adult life. However, it is likely that most of these adults will still have a tendency towards asthma and they should be aware that any recurrence of respiratory symptoms in later life may well be due to asthma.

Any adult who develops cough, wheezing, shortness of breath or chest tightness that is episodic and that may follow a cold or other trigger exposure may well have asthma – and probably does if they had asthma as a child.

Asthma can occur *de novo* at any age. The childhood asthmatic who has 'grown out of it' is especially vulnerable as they may deny that the recurrence of their symptoms could possibly be due to asthma. They may therefore ignore the symptoms and seek help or intervention at a late stage.

The differential diagnosis is of upper or lower respiratory tract infections, postnasal drip, pneumothorax, heart failure, sarcoidosis or tuberculosis. *See Q. 2.4 and Q. 2.36*

5.41   What triggers are relevant when managing asthma in adults?

Triggers that were important in childhood asthma may not necessarily be the same ones that are implicated in the later re-emergence of symptoms. Cigarette smoke should be avoided by everybody, but especially those adults who had childhood asthma.

Triggers are, as always, usually identified by taking a careful history. Skin prick tests can occasionally be useful. Most adult-onset asthma is intrinsic rather than atopic. Anti-house dust mite measures are much less likely to be helpful in adult-onset asthma.

5.42   What medication should I use for adults with asthma?

All adult asthmatics require an inhaled short-acting bronchodilator and they nearly all require regularly inhaled steroids ($<$ 800 µg/day). Many will also require regular inhaled long-acting β_2-agonists. A minority also require one or more of the following:

- Oral LTRAs
- High-dose inhaled steroids (800–2000 µg/day)
- Oral theophyllines
- Oral long-acting β_2-agonists.

The choice of inhaler device depends greatly on the individual patient, but most adults are capable of using most devices. MDIs are the cheapest and are the universal device, but not all asthmatics can use them perfectly.

5.43 Should adult asthmatics have a management plan?

All should have a basic action plan so that they know how to recognize deterioration, how and when to alter their own management, and how and when to call for help. Some will need a more complex, written agreed plan (see *Figs 4.2 and 4.3*).

All will require a good understanding of their disorder and its management in order to achieve perfect control and good compliance. Good education is again the key.

All asthmatics should be reviewed at least annually when their self-management plan should be revised and agreed, and their inhaler technique checked.

5.44 When should I refer an adult with asthma?

If:

- There is diagnostic uncertainty
- The asthma is proving difficult to control
- Long-term high-dose inhaled steroids are being contemplated
- There is significant co-morbidity (such as heart disease, other respiratory diseases, metabolic disorder).

ASTHMA MANAGEMENT IN PREGNANCY

5.45 What happens to asthma in pregnancy?

Asthma is a common condition affecting people of all ages, including women of reproductive age. Pregnancy is also common, especially in women aged between 15 and 45 years. It follows that many asthmatics will get pregnant. If a pregnant woman who is a known asthmatic develops respiratory symptoms in pregnancy, the chances are that the symptoms are due to asthma. However, care must be taken that the woman has not got left ventricular failure or pneumonia, either of which need prompt and proper treatment, and can cause problems for the mother and fetus if adequate treatment is delayed. Valvular heart disease may only become apparent for the first time during pregnancy as a result of the extra cardiovascular strains that the condition imposes.

Some asthmatic women will find that pregnancy worsens their asthma, some that it improves it, and some that it makes no difference.

5.46 What triggers are relevant when managing asthma in pregnancy?

The triggers for asthmatic pregnant women are no different than for other asthmatics. It may well be that trigger avoidance during pregnancy by mothers whose babies are at a high risk of developing asthma may be particularly beneficial, especially if the trigger avoidance continues for the baby after birth.

5.47 What medication should I use for pregnant women with asthma?

All the drugs used to treat asthma, which are given by inhalation in usual doses, are completely safe right through pregnancy, from preconception until the puerperium. The dangers to the fetus of poorly controlled asthma, and especially of hypoxia, far outweigh any problems with any of the drugs.

Even the use of systemic corticosteroids has not been shown to cause great problems, unless taken in high dosage throughout the pregnancy or as frequent courses, when they may be associated with decreased birthweight of the baby. However, this risk is probably less dangerous than the possible hypoxia that may result from poorly controlled asthma.

High-dose β_2-agonists can inhibit uterine contractions, but this is not clinically relevant if they are given by inhalation. There are too few data to establish the safety of leukotriene receptor antagonists in pregnancy or with breast-feeding.

If possible, avoid oral medication, especially oral long-acting β_2-agonists and theophyllines.

5.48 Should pregnant asthmatics have a management plan?

Self-management plans should be agreed and followed in pregnant women in exactly the same way as if the woman was not pregnant. If anything, the threshold for increasing therapy should be lowered, as it is better to overtreat than to undertreat asthma during pregnancy. Obviously, inhaler technique and the self-management plan should be reviewed throughout the pregnancy and puerperium.

Patients with inadequate inhaled anti-inflammatory treatment during pregnancy run a higher risk of suffering an acute attack of asthma than those receiving treatment with an adequate dose of anti-inflammatory agent. If an acute attack of asthma should occur, prompt and early treatment does not have serious affects on the pregnancy, delivery or health of the newborn infant.

Breast-feeding should make no difference to the type or quantity of medication.

5.49 When should I refer a pregnant woman with asthma?

The management of pregnant asthmatics should be along the same lines as that for non-pregnant women. Advice may be needed from a respiratory physician and obstetrician from time to time. The midwife must also be involved, and she has a key role in reinforcing the importance of compliance with preventive treatment, and in promptly recognizing and treating any deterioration. It is important to continue treatment in the puerperium.

MANAGING BRITTLE ASTHMA

5.50 What is brittle asthma and how can I diagnose it?

Brittle asthma refers to asthma in patients who suffer repeated life-threatening asthma attacks. There are two types of brittle asthma:

- ■ *Type 1* – Such patients have recurrent asthma attacks on a background of widely variable peak flow readings (more than 40% diurnal variation on most days) despite maximal medical therapy. Type 1 brittle asthma is three times more common in women than in men. Many patients have complex psychosocial problems and have often experienced sexual or physical abuse. Some patients may hyperventilate in response to worsening asthma.
- ■ *Type 2* – Such patients suffer an attack of asthma that becomes severe within minutes or hours, despite having little instability in their asthma in the preceding days or weeks. Indeed, such patients may have absolutely no symptoms attributable to asthma in the interim, and may have steady and good peak flow readings. This type is equally common in men and women, and there is not usually any underlying psychiatric or psychological morbidity.

Type 1 brittle asthma is more common than type 2, but both types are rare. The diagnosis is based solely on the history and peak flow readings.

5.51 What triggers are relevant when managing brittle asthma?

Patients with type 1 brittle asthma are usually strongly atopic but choose not to avoid any allergens. They usually smoke and keep dogs and other pets.

Triggers in patients with type 2 brittle asthma can be difficult to identify, but if identified they should be avoided vigorously.

Skin prick testing may be particularly useful in these patients. They need to avoid any likely triggers and, if such triggers can be shown to be more likely by skin prick testing, this will help with more specific avoidance. Of course, such avoidance may not always be practical, or possible.

5.52 What medication should I use in patients with brittle asthma?
TYPE 1

Patients will often be on many drugs, many at high or heroic doses, including high-dose, long-term oral steroids. The patients often change the doses of all or some of their drugs, not necessarily logically or in proportion to their symptoms or peak flow readings (which are often not taken). Drugs and doses should be reviewed regularly and the dosage of oral steroids kept to the minimum necessary. Continuous subcutaneous terbutaline may rarely be of help, preferably after an inpatient double-blind trial with clearly defined objective criteria of efficacy. Respiratory physiotherapy may help with control of breathing, as may relaxation exercises.

TYPE 2

Patients should always have an easily accessible supply of a suitable bronchodilator inhaler, which they are happy and able to use. Ideally they should also have a large-volume spacer available. In addition they should have a supply of oral steroids, preferably not enteric-coated, for emergency use. They may need duplicate supplies of the bronchodilator inhalers and the oral steroids so that they have access at home, at work and, for instance, in the car. A Medic-Alert bracelet or equivalent is a good idea.

5.53 Should patients with brittle asthma have a management plan?

TYPE 1

These patients often react erratically and inconsistently to events and are poor at anticipating or predicting deterioration. Written self-management plans should regularly be reviewed and agreed. Some form of bargaining and subsequent contract-making between patient and clinician should be attempted. Criteria for self-admission need to be agreed with the patient and hospital.

TYPE 2

The patient's chronic asthma must be optimally managed at all times. At the first inkling of the beginning of an attack, the patient should call for help. He or she should then immediately take high-dose inhaled short-acting β_2-agonists, ideally 20–50 puffs via a large-volume spacer, or 5 mg via a nebulizer. The patient should also take 30–60 mg prednisolone immediately and go straight to the nearest hospital.

If previous attacks have been very severe, the patient should self-inject adrenaline subcutaneously or intramuscularly, having been previously instructed on how to do this by the practice nurse or general practitioner, and attend the nearest accident and emergency department, even if there is apparently full recovery. The patient will need to be monitored fairly regularly, and their ability to recognize the early signs and to respond promptly should be regularly revised.

5.54 When should I refer a patient with brittle asthma?

All patients with brittle asthma should be managed jointly by the primary healthcare team and a respiratory physician. The patient's family, carers and colleagues at work should all be aware that the patient may have sudden catastrophic asthma and they should know how best to help. In some cases this may mean just calling the ambulance and allowing the patient to administer their own medication; in other cases help may be needed in injecting adrenaline or using a nebulizer.

Type 1 brittle asthma sufferers have complex problems. Medical management is often complicated by poor compliance. Management must be holistic, with attention paid to the roles of diet (often low in vitamins A, C and E, and in trace elements) and exercise. Psychological help is often needed, but not always wanted.

Brittle asthma, understandably, is the cause of great anxiety to patients and their relatives and carers.

MANAGING MIXED OBSTRUCTIVE AIRWAY DISEASE

5.55 What is mixed obstructive airway disease?

This phrase describes patients who have a mixture of chronic obstructive pulmonary disease (COPD) (either emphysema, chronic bronchitis or both) and asthma. 'Pure' COPD implies airway obstruction that is irreversible, as opposed to the reversible or partially reversible airway obstruction that occurs in asthma. In practice, many patients will have a mixture of COPD and asthma. Such patients are often said to have partially reversible COPD. There is considerable overlap between COPD and asthma.

5.56 How can I diagnose mixed obstructive airway disease?

COPD has been defined as a chronic, slowly progressive, disease characterized by reduced maximum expiratory flow and slow forced emptying of the lungs – features that do not change markedly over several months. Airflow obstruction is relatively fixed but bronchodilator therapy may result in some improvement. COPD normally comes on in late middle age and affects men more than women. In the UK nowadays it is a common complication of smoking, and is rarely seen in lifelong non-smokers. The breathlessness and coughing is usually insidious in onset and is far less episodic than 'pure' asthma. With COPD, there will be not only reduced peak flow readings but also reduced FEV_1 readings. Even after treatment with inhaled bronchodilators or oral steroids, FEV_1 or peak flow readings will not return to their theoretical normal value, and the improvement will be less than 15%. With COPD extensive pulmonary damage has usually occurred before a patient is aware of any symptoms. The structural changes that occur in the lungs in COPD are irreversible, although their progress can be slowed or halted. This is in contrast to 'pure' asthma, where the anatomical changes in the lungs are far less marked and are less likely to be permanent unless the asthma has been poorly treated or is very severe over a long period of time.

The symptoms of COPD may mimic those of asthma. Both can cause wheezing, shortness of breath, chest tightness and cough. In asthma, however, the symptoms are usually paroxysmal or episodic and are often worse at night, whereas in COPD they tend to be much more chronic, usually begin with exertional breathlessness and morning cough, and do not usually affect sleep. The differential diagnosis between these two disorders can be difficult, and there is often some degree of overlap. The main differentiating feature between COPD and asthma is the lack of reversibility in peak flow or FEV_1 in response to treatment. *See Q. 2.39.*

5.57 What triggers are relevant when managing mixed obstructive airway disease?

COPD is caused almost exclusively by cigarette smoking. Cigarette smoking can certainly exacerbate asthma and make the asthma more difficult to control. Patients with COPD who give up smoking will prevent further decline in lung function and further anatomical deterioration in the lungs.

Common triggers in mixed obstructive airway disease are the same as those for asthma. Exercise is normally a very potent trigger, as is cold air. Dust and smoky atmospheres may exacerbate the airway obstruction, but exposure to house dust mite and other allergens is rarely of clinical importance.

5.58 What medication should I use in mixed obstructive airway disease?

- Patients with mixed obstructive airway disease nearly always benefit from regular bronchodilators taken by inhalation.
- Anticholinergics are more useful for patients with mixed obstructive airway disease in many cases, because the cholinergic tone is the main reversible component in COPD. There is often an additive effect between anticholinergics and short-acting β_2-agonists.
- Long-acting β_2-agonists can be of help for persistent night-time or exercise-induced symptoms where some reversibility has been demonstrated.
- Theophyllines may help some patients.
- Nearly all patients with mixed obstructive airway disease benefit from the regular use of inhaled steroids. A steroid trial should be given and the FEV_1 and peak flow should be measured before the trial begins. A 3 week course of high-dose steroid should be given and respiratory

function monitored during and after the course. If there has been an improvement in the peak flow or FEV_1 of more than 20%, the management should be as for asthma. If there is no reversibility and the patient does not feel any symptomatic improvement, there is little point in continuing with the inhaled steroids and the patient should be managed as for COPD. If there is objective improvement of FEV_1 or peak flow of > 20%, and the patient feels symptomatically better, long-term inhaled steroid therapy may be justified. However, no effect from long-term inhaled steroids on lung function and responsiveness will be usual.

■ The best device for people with mixed obstructive airway disease is one that they are able and happy to use.

■ Large-volume spacers are often the most efficient way of delivering treatment for patients with COPD.

■ Trials of nebulization should be given only when all other inhaler devices have not produced maximal symptomatic or peak flow improvements, and only when monitored by regular peak flow (preferably) FEV_1 measurements. Failure of improvement in the FEV_1 despite regular nebulizations probably means that their continuation is an unjustified expense.

■ *See Q. 2.40*

5.59 Should patients with mixed obstructive airway disease have a management plan?

Patients with mixed obstructive airway disease should receive the same education, support and follow-up as patients with 'pure' asthma. Compliance with therapy, and especially with giving up smoking, is very important. These patients may need antibiotics for acute infective exacerbations.

5.60 When should I refer patients with mixed obstructive airway disease, or should I manage them in my asthma clinic?

Patients with an asthmatic component to their COPD should receive the care similar to those with 'pure' asthma. There are now good guidelines for the management of COPD,[12] and patients with 'pure' COPD should *not* be seen in the asthma clinic. The poor response of these patients to therapy can be dispiriting to those setting up asthma clinics and to the patients themselves and their families. However, they should receive appropriate care and follow-up from within both primary and secondary care.

Although it may be inappropriate to manage patients with COPD in the asthma clinic, do not dismiss them completely. A diagnosis of emphysema or chronic bronchitis is usually not well received and such patients' self-esteem and self-confidence can be further demoralized if they are told that their illness is all their own fault for smoking. It is important to remove such patients from the asthma clinic tactfully and to offer alternative care, support and management, preferably from within the primary heathcare setting.

Good management of patients with mixed obstructive airway disease is challenging. Many patients will be also under the care of a respiratory physician, especially those who may require or who have required hospital admissions for acute exacerbations.

MANAGING OCCUPATIONAL ASTHMA

5.61 What is meant by occupational asthma?

Occupational asthma is asthma due to causes and conditions attributable to the particular occupational environment and not commonly found outside the workplace. Thus occupational asthma excludes bronchoconstriction induced by irritants such as exercise and cold air, even though these may also be encountered at work. *See also Q. 1.14.*

5.62 How common is it?

Occupational asthma is the most common occupational respiratory ailment, and accounts for about 25% of all such cases. There are two main forms. The first is when asthma occurs after a latent period of exposure, and the second when there is no such latency but usually in response to a high concentration of irritant. Between 2% and 6% of workers will be affected, which corresponds to about 50 cases per million working people per year.

The epidemiology of occupational lung disease in Britain has been greatly enhanced by the Surveillance of Work-related and Occupational Respiratory Disease (SWORD) Project, which was established in 1989 and is sponsored by the Health and Safety Executive. Occupational and respiratory physicians are invited to report new cases of occupational lung disease with the suspected agents. The data are analysed and the results published annually.[13]

5.63 What are the most common causes of occupational asthma?

In the UK there are more than 200 known respiratory sensitizers, and more are identified each year. Some sensitizers may not be immediately obvious. The major causes of occupational asthma and the groups at risk are shown in *Table 1.1.* The causative agents are listed in descending order of frequency.

5.64　How can I diagnose occupational asthma?

The diagnosis is based on the history. A detailed and comprehensive occupational history is essential in the initial assessment of anyone thought to have occupational asthma. The first symptom is often coughing at the end of a shift. Symptoms generally improve at weekends and holidays, but at a later stage the symptoms may persist all the time. Further examination is rarely helpful. Serial peak flow measurements may help with the diagnosis.

Skin prick tests can occasionally be helpful. Liaison with a company's occupational health physician, if there is one, may also be helpful to the patient.

A fall in peak respiratory flow rates or substantial diurnal variability on working days but not on days away from work supports a diagnosis of occupational asthma. Patients often experience symptoms that are worse on Mondays, often recovering by the end of the week as they adapt; other patients find that their symptoms build up during the week and are at their worst on Thursday, often being unable to return to work on Fridays. If there is any doubt about the diagnosis, the patient should be referred to a respiratory physician. If the diagnosis is clear-cut, the patient should be referred to an occupational or respiratory physician for confirmation. The ultimate test is a bronchial challenge.

5.65　How should I manage occupational asthma?

The asthma should be managed as usual. However, it is important to be aware that, once somebody has been sensitized to a specific substance, subsequent exposure even to tiny amounts of that substance may precipitate severe acute asthma.

Anybody who develops occupational asthma should avoid any further exposure to the causative agent. This may mean relocation or loss of current employment, so it is important to identify the specific cause accurately.

Occupational asthma is a prescribed occupational disease in the UK. A worker who develops the condition is entitled to 'no fault' compensation if the degree of disability is 14% or more. Further details are available in the Department of Social Services leaflet *Occupational Asthma* (Ref NI237). Benefit is not taxable, not income-related and non-contributory. Claims should be made using form B1100-OA. It is advisable to refer patients to a chest physician first (to confirm the diagnosis of occupational asthma).

> Another approach is to eliminate totally the exposure of the individual to the suspect agent whilst remaining in the same employment. This is not always feasible.
>
> In view of the implications on unemployment, some patients are reluctant to accept that they may have asthma, much less that their asthma may be occupationally related.
>
> All patients with suspected occupational asthma should be referred for assessment by a respiratory specialist.

5.66 What about a career in the armed forces for asthmatic patients?

Until recently, asthma was a bar to joining HM forces in the UK. Nowadays, a past history of asthma is not necessarily a bar. Entry will not be denied if the asthma was mild and there have been no acute episodes in the previous two years and no need for treatment in that time.

Should asthma occur in a person already in the forces, they may well be redeployed in UK-based units or advised against certain occupations or active service. However, such a diagnosis no longer means that the patient is automatically considered unfit to remain as a serving member of the forces.

MANAGING ASTHMA IN THE ELDERLY

5.67 How can I diagnose asthma in this age group?

Asthma can start at any age: the elderly are not exempt. Asthma is probably underdiagnosed in the elderly as it is mistaken for either COPD or heart failure. Another reason for the diagnosis being overlooked and the disease subsequently being undertreated is older people's tolerance of respiratory symptoms.

There is also some evidence to suggest that elderly people with asthma have a lower perception of a given degree of airway narrowing than younger people experiencing the same degree of narrowing. However, the airways of elderly asthmatics are as sensitive as those of younger patients, and elderly asthmatics should not be undertreated.

Generally, elderly people welcome a diagnosis that not only explains their symptoms but for which there are good, effective and safe treatments.

Conditions to consider in the differential diagnosis are COPD, bronchiectasis and congestive cardiac failure, all of which may be indistinguishable from asthma by the history alone. New respiratory symptoms in middle-aged or elderly smokers, or ex-smokers, may be due to lung cancer; so have a very low threshold for requesting a chest radiograph in such patients, and refer to a chest physician if there is any doubt regarding the true diagnosis of asthma. *See Q. 2.5 and Q. 2.37*

5.68 What triggers are relevant when managing asthma in the elderly?

Most asthma in the elderly is intrinsic and triggered by upper respiratory tract infection, exercise or cold air. Allergen identification and avoidance is not usually very fruitful. Smoking should, as for all asthmatics, be avoided.

5.69 What medication should I use in elderly patients with asthma?

The principles of management are the same as for younger adults (*see Q. 5.42*).

■ Many elderly patients will benefit from long-acting inhaled bronchodilators to help their night symptoms or exercise-induced symptoms.
■ Oral bronchodilators and/or theophyllines should be avoided as first-line therapies because they are more likely to induce side-effects or have unwanted interactions with other medications the elderly patient may be taking.
■ Many elderly people have difficulty with coordination, and many suffer from poor sight or arthritis affecting the hands. For these reasons, elderly patients should be given the opportunity to try out various different types of inhaler and to use the ones they feel happiest with. Metered-dose inhalers are frequently unsuitable. However, large-volume spacers with metered-dose inhalers are probably the treatment of choice, especially if high-dose inhaled steroids are needed.

5.70 Should elderly asthmatics have a management plan?

The elderly require education and understanding in a similar fashion to patients in all other age groups. Compliance and inhaler technique needs to be checked, especially if other faculties are failing.

5.71 When should I refer elderly patients with asthma?

The successful management of asthma in the elderly can usually be provided from within primary care. In the infirm elderly, the help of family, nursing home staff or day-carers may also be needed. It is important that everybody tries to aim for perfection in managing the elderly, just as they would for people at all other ages, and referral should follow the same criteria as for younger adults (*see Q. 5.44*).

MANAGING DIFFICULT ASTHMA

5.72   A few of my patients seem to have troublesome symptoms and sudden changes in asthma control despite small falls in their peak flow readings. Why is this and how should I manage them?

A number of asthmatic patients seem to be very high perceivers of minimal change to their airway calibre and they also tend to respond by inappropriate hyperventilation. This leads to worsening dyspnoea, increased anxiety, and the use of high doses of medication. Increasing anxiety levels lead to an increased ability to detect small changes in airway obstruction. These patients tend to be high attenders both at their GP's surgery and at hospital emergency and outpatient departments, and are frequently admitted to hospital. They take and need a lot of time. Simple reassurance is not helpful. They need a careful explanation of their disease and that they are in a subgroup whose responses are oversensitive, through no fault of their own. They will need to be given the confidence to manage their own asthma in a logical way without panicking. This is not a simple neurosis, although many patients will be generally anxious. Patients will need detailed, agreed, self-management plans (peak flow led rather than symptom led). Although relaxation and biofeedback therapies are generally ineffective in asthma management, this small group of patients may benefit from such approaches.

5.73   I also have a few patients who don't seem to appreciate that their asthma has become very severe until quite late. How can I help them?

In a similar vein to the answer above, a number of asthmatics seem to be low perceivers of quite marked changes in their airway. Some patients will be subconsciously in denial of their disease and the need to control it, but others will be well motivated. These patients seek help late and are at an increased risk of dying from severe asthma. They are a difficult group to manage. Regular peak flow readings, even when feeling well, are strongly advised, with peak flow-led self-management plans combined with education and regular follow-up. These patients need to be motivated to monitor their asthma and to increase their self-management, even when feeling well.

COMPLIANCE

5.74 One of the biggest problems I have is getting my patients to comply with the suggested management. Why is this and how can I improve compliance?

It is a source of great disappointment and occasional amazement that, despite the best efforts of doctors and nurses, patients fail to comply with the excellent and logical treatment regimens presented to them. Non-compliance is especially a problem with regular preventive treatment in asthma, and has been estimated to be as high as 50%.[14] Many factors contribute to non-compliance, including misunderstandings about the disease and its treatment, underestimating expectations about the efficacy of treatment, and lack of knowledge about the different roles of preventer and reliever treatments. Non-compliance is a particular problem with inhaled therapies, and does not appear to be a problem only for inhaled steroids. Correlations with good compliance include the perception by the patient that the drug is useful, and the perception of the drug regimen as regular. Better compliance also correlates with low frequency of dosage, and whether the patient has seen a specialist. Compliance is increased with symptoms that would otherwise occur daily.

Modern synonyms include adherence or concordance.

5.75 Is poor compliance just due to patients' ignorance?

Factors affecting non-compliance include patient concerns about their disease, about acute attacks and about the side-effects of drugs. This is especially true when considering fear or misunderstanding of inhaled steroids. Patients may also have concerns about the stigma of being labelled asthmatic; refusal to accept the diagnosis will result in poor compliance with therapy. In general, patients who find treatment logical and easy to use, and without side-effects (either real or perceived), are more likely to comply with therapy than those who are taking the drugs because their therapist tells them to. Indeed, education alone has little effect on compliance, whereas combining education with training and behavioural therapy will show improvement in compliance and in the quality of patients' lives.

5.76 Are there different types of non-compliance?

Non-compliance is either deliberate or accidental:

■ *Deliberate* non-compliance results from the patient's beliefs regarding the cause of their asthma, how serious it is, the likely benefits and costs of therapy, their past experiences and their relationship with the doctor or nurse. Many patients feel that they will lose control of their lives and their asthma by complying with therapy suggested by other people, including the nurse or doctor. Patients react emotionally and intellectually to changes, and often the emotion will dominate the intellectual response. Many type 1 brittle asthmatics fit this model.

■ *Accidental* non-compliance is less common but more straightforward. Patients may fail to understand what has been discussed with them because of poor concentration (often due to anxiety or depression), poor memory, poor comprehension (especially if their English is poor), poor intellect, or perhaps they are just scatterbrained!

The Impact of Asthma Survey[7] found that 45% of respondents admitted that they did not exactly follow the instructions given to them for taking their medication. The commonest reasons given were that they took only the medication that they felt they needed, or that they simply forgot, or they felt better, or they thought the medication was not really necessary anyway. The same survey cited nearly half of respondents as wanting more information about treatment, so the lesson of better and more appropriate education seems clear.

5.77 How can I improve my patients' compliance?

Recommendations for improving compliance should include the following:

■ Simple drug regimens
■ Handwritten instructions
■ Good patient–doctor or patient–nurse rapport
■ Minimization of possible side-effects
■ Patient education.

The most important factors contributing to non-compliance with asthma medication are lack of knowledge about the disease and the need for long-term maintenance therapy even in the absence of symptoms.

5.78 How can I get my patients to take their inhaled steroids?

In general practice, poor compliance with inhaled steroid therapy is common. Generally, the media are ignorant about inhaled steroids and readily broadcast misinformed or sensational negative reports. These can cause untold damage to many patients' confidence and may undermine the hard work done by many doctors and nurses over many years.

To improve compliance, it may be useful to educate patients as follows:

■ Acknowledge that asthma inhibits growth: the more severe and more poorly controlled the asthma, the greater the effect on growth retardation. This effect is also seen in children with eczema, so it may reflect some fundamental property of atopy rather than of asthma itself.

■ Asthma can delay maturation, and this is true especially if the asthma is poorly controlled and inhaled steroids have never been used. This may also be an atopy-related phenomenon. The delay is not usual and, if it occurs, is not critical.

■ Systemic steroids inhibit growth and development. It is for these reasons that inhaled steroids were developed.

■ Inhaled steroids have dose-related systemic effects, but the systemic absorption of inhaled steroids is negligible if given in normal doses. Even when given in higher doses, there is occasionally biochemical evidence of dose-related adrenal suppression, which is rarely clinically important.

■ Emphasize that the adult height for asthmatic children is normal, regardless of whether or not they had inhaled steroids at whatever dose during childhood.

SMOKING AND ASTHMA

5.79   Is smoking a problem in asthma?

Smoking is undoubtedly a harmful habit for everybody who indulges. It is especially harmful for those who already have lung diseases such as asthma. Although not a cause of asthma, smoking is a frequent cause of exacerbations of asthma at all ages. Babies with an asthmatic tendency (those with a strong family history of atopy and asthma) are more likely to develop asthma in later life if their mother smoked during pregnancy or if exposed to second-hand cigarette smoke during the first year of life.

All doctors and nurses working in primary care have a duty to try to help all their asthmatic smokers to stop smoking, and to protect all asthmatics from the effects of second-hand cigarette smoke. In a few cases simple education and pointing out the facts will be sufficient. However, smoking is an addictive habit that many people find difficult to give up. Coupled with the addiction may be feelings of guilt. Patients may be economical with the truth when admitting to their habits or to the extent of their habits – and certainly to their behaviour in front of their children.

5.80 How can I help my patients stop smoking?

Better approaches are required than simply pointing out the evils of smoking. It is better to get patients to agree that they want not to smoke and actively want to stop. This may take time and patience. To achieve these goals it is best not to alienate the smoker but to help him or her agree that they have a problem that they would like to overcome and that can be overcome – although admittedly not always easily. Most primary care trusts in England and Wales have a smoking cessation clinic to which patients can be referred.

Helping asthmatic patients who smoke to give up smoking is a challenge for all doctors and nurses along with asthma care. It is not an optional role.

MANAGING ASTHMA IN PATIENTS WITH OTHER DISEASES

5.81 Many of my asthma patients have other disorders. Will their asthma management be different?

UPPER AIRWAY DISEASE

Asthma is often associated with rhinitis, sinusitis and nasal polyps. Proper attention to these conditions and correct treatment will facilitate effective asthma management, and may be an essential prerequisite for the management of some people's asthma.

PSYCHOSOCIAL FACTORS

Asthma may cause anxiety and depression in sufferers and their carers. Asthma and psychological or psychiatric illness can obviously coexist without one being a cause of the other. The mortality rate from asthma is increased by depression, alcohol abuse, unemployment, schizophrenia, bereavement and family disruption. There is some evidence to suggest that non-compliance with treatment may be common in those with depression and that psychosocial problems may have been commoner in those who have died from asthma. Patients who use major tranquillizers and who also have asthma are more likely to suffer increased illness and death. *See Q. 1.18, Q. 5.72 and Q. 5.73.*

GASTRO-OESOPHAGEAL REFLUX DISEASE (GORD)

Asthma and GORD often occur together, each exacerbating the other. Good control of either condition helps to control the other, or may be a prerequisite.

EXERCISE-INDUCED ASTHMA

5.82 What is exercise-induced asthma?

Exercise is a common trigger of asthma; in some asthmatics it is the only one. The inability to exercise normally is often underestimated by patient and doctor alike. Exercise-induced asthma symptoms occur in about 70–80% of all asthmatics.

The exact mechanism by which exercise induces bronchoconstriction is not clear. It is probably caused by the increased ventilation that always occurs on exercise, resulting in inadequately warmed and inadequately humidified air reaching the lungs. Thus, exercise results in the inhalation of relatively dry and cold air, and this is thought to be more important than the metabolic changes caused by exercise itself. Exercise-induced asthma is typically present 5–15 minutes after exercise, and may last for up to an hour. There may be an additional late response up to 10 hours later.

Exercise-induced asthma may be a mark of poorly controlled asthma; better overall control of the asthma may result in better control of the exercise-induced symptoms. Some people may have normal lung function and good control of their asthma most of the time, and have symptoms only when exercising or active.

Symptoms may be induced by different degrees of activity in different people. At worst, everyday activities may bring on asthma symptoms, such as children playing normally with their friends or adults doing tasks of daily living such as vacuuming or cleaning the car. Other people may get symptoms only when participating in sport. Finally, there may be competitive athletes for whom even minor changes of asthma control may affect their performance. Bear in mind that many asthmatics may have low expectations of their ability to exercise and therefore have self-imposed restrictions.

Not everybody who has exercise-induced coughing, wheezing and breathlessness has necessarily got exercise-induced asthma. They may just be generally unfit, or have cardiac disease or other respiratory disease. Identification of those with true exercise-induced asthma can be made by regular peak flow monitoring before and after exercise. A fall in peak flow of more than 20% up to 20 minutes after cessation of exercise is diagnostic of exercise-induced asthma. *See also Q. 1.11.*

5.83 How can I diagnose exercise-induced asthma?

It is important to ask the right questions to the right patients:

- In *children*, the doctor or nurse needs to ask whether the child joins in with their peer group at play, and whether their teachers notice any problems with sport or exercise. Are they able to join in formal sport at school or do they, for example, always play the goalkeeper or wicketkeeper? Do they prefer playing indoors or outdoors?

■ In *adolescents*, the doctor or nurse needs to ask whether they take regular exercise and, if so, whether they enjoy it. Do they shy away from activities where they might be embarrassed by their inability to perform or participate?

■ In *adults*, what exercise do they undertake and are these exercises limited because of their asthma? If they do not take exercise is it because they are frightened that the asthma may be provoked?

■ In *sportsmen and women*, what sports are most likely to trigger the asthma, and does this affect their ability to compete or train? Is their level of proficiency impaired?

5.84 How should I manage exercise-induced asthma?

The management of exercise-induced asthma involves the following non-pharmaceutical measures:

■ The doctor or nurse should encourage full physical fitness.

■ The patient should avoid triggers such as smoking and, if possible, cold air, and any known allergens.

■ Sports less likely to provoke asthma include swimming and steady indoor exercise in a warm moist environment.

■ Committed athletes should be advised to use steady warm-up exercises in advance of their event and if possible to avoid cold dry environments.

■ Before turning to pharmacological measures for exercise-induced asthma, it is important to establish that the asthma is well controlled apart from during exercise or activity. Consider, as always, compliance with medication and inhaler technique.

■ Premedication is the mainstay of treatment for symptoms induced by exercise. Unpredictable activity may occur especially in children, and this will influence the choice of therapy.

5.85 What medications are useful in exercise-induced asthma?

The following therapies may be considered:

■ *Inhaled short-acting β_2-agonists* given 15–30 minutes before exercise. The effects should last between 4 and 6 hours, and provide acute relief or prevention of exercise-induced symptoms. They are useful for people who experience only occasional symptoms because they provide rapid relief.

■ *Inhaled long-acting β_2-agonists*. These last for up to 12 hours and can be given on the morning of a day that will involve multiple bouts of exercise. They are also useful for children when exercise may be unpredictable, when they can be given once or twice every day. A short-acting bronchodilator may also be necessary for acute relief. Regular use of long-acting β_2-agonists should not be given in the absence of other anti-inflammatory treatment.

■ *Oral LTRAs* given regularly, or intermittently. The effect lasts for 24 hours and comes on within a few hours of taking the dose, so a tablet can be taken the night before a football game or athletics competition, for example, or LTRAs can be used in the same way as inhaled long-acting β_2-agonists.

■ *Sodium cromoglicate or nedocromil.* These drugs are best given 30 minutes before exercise; they have few side-effects. A short-acting inhaled bronchodilator may also be necessary.

■ *Ipratropium bromide* is best given 30–60 minutes before exercise. It is useful if short-acting bronchodilators do not appear to control symptoms. Ipratropium may not provide such rapid relief as short-acting inhaled bronchodilators, so the latter may also be needed for acute relief.

5.86 What about longer-term management and prevention of exercise-induced asthma?

Particular attention should be paid to the good control of asthma. The regular use of inhaled steroids for two months or more reduces the incidence of exercise-induced asthma and the severity of exercise-induced symptoms. However, even if the asthma is generally well controlled, exercise-induced symptoms may still occur. Exercise is an important part of most people's lives, especially children. One of the goals of asthma management is to allow people to be involved in normal activity, including full participation in exercise or sport. This goal is attainable in most patients.

5.87 What about professional or representative sports – are there any problems with taking asthma medications?

Most prescribed treatments for asthma are allowed in competitive sports, but those competing at national or international levels should check with their individual sports or with the British Olympic Association.

Table 5.5 lists the substances and drugs permitted or prohibited by the International Olympic Committee, but it is always wise to check with each sport's governing body, or with the UK Sport Drug Information Line +44 (0) 20 7841 9530.

TABLE 5.5 Medication allowed or banned by the British Olympic Association

Condition	Drugs allowed	Drugs banned
Asthma*	Cromogens Salbutamol Terbutaline Salmeterol Formoterol (eformoterol) Beclometasone Budesonide Fluticasone Theophyllines	All products containing sympathomimetics, e.g. ephedrine, isoprenaline, fenoterol, rimiterol, orciprenaline
Cough	All antibiotics Menthol inhalations Terfenadine Astemizole Pholcodine Dextromethorphan Guaipenesin Paracetamol	Products containing sympathomimetics: Ephedrine Pseudoephedrine Phenylpropanolamine
Hay fever	Terfenadine Astemizole Cromoglicate eye-drops Nasal sprays containing steroids or xylometazoline	As for cough

* These drugs are allowed if given by inhalation (except theophyllines) and written notification of administration has been given to the relevant medical authority

5.88 Surely asthma must be a handicap at some levels of sport?

At higher levels, well-managed asthma is no bar to success: 41 Olympic medals, including 15 gold and 21 silver medals were won by American athletes suffering from exercise induced-asthma during the 1992 Summer Olympics. Asthma has not prevented such stars as Ian Botham, Steve Ovett, Paul Scholes and Ian Wright from reaching the top of their sporting trees.

MANAGING TROUBLESOME SYMPTOMS

5.89 What is cough variant asthma?

Patients who present only with coughing, usually worse on exertion and at night, present a diagnostic dilemma. In children, asthma is the most likely explanation for chronic or persistent dry cough, especially if the cough is worse during the night. In adults with persistent or recurrent cough, chest radiography is advisable after a full history and examination. The main differential diagnoses and their tests include:

- *Cough-variant asthma*: spirometry, peak flow charts, trials of treatment.
- *Chronic nasal catarrh and postnasal drip*: examination, computed tomography of the sinuses, referral to an ear, nose and throat department.
- *Gastro-oesophageal reflux*: trial of a proton pump inhibitor for two months (at maximum dosage); endoscopy or barium studies.
- *Bronchiectasis, tuberculosis, lung cancer*: chest radiography, computed tomography of thorax.
- *No cause found*: in about a third of patients with a chronic dry cough, no cause can be found. Referral to a chest physician is indicated if the primary care physician is unable to find a cause.

5.90 What should I do if the asthma seems to be persistently worse at night?

Asthma that is worse at night may be due to poor underlying control. Serial peak flow measurements are required, as well as a symptom diary. Medication that is particularly useful at night, and that can be used in addition to regular inhaled steroids, includes inhaled long-acting β_2-agonists, oral LTRAs and oral slow-release theophyllines. Theophyllines are most likely to cause side-effects and should be tried last.

New or re-emerging night symptoms are often the first warning of loss of asthma control, and may develop into acute severe asthma. Treat the re-emergence of night symptoms promptly and aggressively with high-dose bronchodilators and possibly a short course of oral steroids.

5.91 What is the role of respiratory infections? Many of my asthmatic patients seem to get chest infections.

One of the most common triggers for asthma is upper respiratory tract infection. These infections are often unavoidable, but at the first symptoms or signs of such an infection asthma therapy should be stepped up. All patients with severe asthma should receive influenza vaccine each autumn, especially those who require long-term high-dose or oral steroids, or more than four courses on average of oral steroids per year. Many patients with upper respiratory tract infection-induced exacerbations of their asthma are wrongly diagnosed as having a chest infection, either by themselves or by their physicians, on the basis of increased symptoms and a productive cough. Green or yellow sputum may indicate increased bronchial inflammation rather than bacterial infection. Antibiotics are usually indicated only if there is fever and purulent or increased sputum, crackles on chest auscultation, or co-morbidity (e.g. bronchiectasis, diabetes). Long-term antibiotic prophylaxis should not be used in managing asthma.

5.92 Should all my asthmatic patients avoid aspirin?

Overall, only about 10% of adults with asthma are thought to be aspirin sensitive, and they are usually people who need chronic treatment with high-dose inhaled steroids. There is probably some cross-reactivity with non-steroidal anti-inflammatory drugs (NSAIDs), but the extent of this and its clinical relevance is not clear. As a general measure, aspirin should be avoided by asthmatics unless they have previously tolerated it without problems. The advice to avoid NSAIDs is also often made on less evidence. Those with a history of aspirin-induced asthma should definitely always avoid aspirin.

■ Patients known to be sensitive should studiously avoid all aspirin and aspirin products, and aspirin-related products such as the NSAIDs (e.g. ibuprofen).

■ Aspirin-sensitive asthma is rarely seen in children (in whom aspirin is contraindicated anyway).

■ Asthmatics who are known not to be aspirin sensitive can safely use aspirin and aspirin-related products.

■ Aspirin-induced asthma has a low correlation with atopy but a higher correlation with chronic rhinitis and nasal polyps.

■ Challenging with aspirin should take place only in hospital when the asthma is in remission.

■ LTRAs are particularly effective in aspirin-sensitive asthma.

See also Q. 1.17 and Q. 4.66.

5.93 Some of my female asthmatic patients say that the severity of their asthma alters with their menstrual cycle. How can I help them?

Some women find that their asthma may be slightly worse at different stages of the menstrual cycle. A good symptom diary together with peak flow readings and a menstrual diary can help to confirm this. A premenstrual increase in symptoms may occur in up to 40% of women with asthma. A few women may find that their asthma worsens during the time of ovulation, or during menstruation.

Premenstrual worsening of asthma may be due to an abnormal level of progesterone during the late luteal phase of menstruation, leading to changes in airway responsiveness in this group of patients. The patients most prone to premenstrual exacerbations are those with severe asthma.

Treatment options are empirical. It is worth doubling the dose of inhaled steroids during the second half of the cycle and/or adding a long-acting β_2-agonist during that time. A logical option would be to add regular oral theophyllines, as there are cyclical changes in airway responsiveness to adenosine monophosphate (AMP), which tends to be highest premenstrually; theophyllines block the adenosine receptors and thus reduce the increase in airway irritability caused by increased AMP levels. A further option might be to consider intramuscular progesterone injections during the late luteal phase in women with severe premenstrual asthma.

If these measures are unsuccessful, refer to a chest physician, who should liaise with an endocrinologist or gynaecologist.

ASTHMA AND TRAVEL

5.94 What advice should I give to asthmatics about travelling?

- On no account should asthmatics stop their preventive medications.
- They should make sure that they have sufficient short-acting bronchodilator or other relievers to last the trip.
- Ideally they should monitor their asthma during their travels by measuring peak flows, and should have a low threshold for using their asthma self-management or action plan and stepping up to the next level of treatment, and for adding in regular short-acting bronchodilators to cover any acute exacerbation at an early stage.
- If past experience indicates that their asthma worsens when visiting particular areas or houses, then the above measures should be started 2–3 days before travelling and continued for that time after returning home.
- Patients should avoid high-altitude holidays, especially if their asthma is severe.
- Skiing is not necessarily contraindicated, but the combination of cold air, exercise and relatively high altitudes provides a potent mix of triggers for many asthmatics. Emphasize the need for good compliance with preventive therapy and action plans, and to increase the amount of exercise gradually in the first few days.

5.95 What advice should I give to asthmatics about flying?

Nearly all patients with asthma are fit to fly on commercial airlines. The following groups of patients need special consideration:

- Those with severe asthma (BTS/SIGN Step 4 or 5; *see Q. 4.95*), especially with dyspnoea at rest.

■ Patients who have had an acute exacerbation requiring admission within the last 6–8 weeks.

■ Patients with co-morbidity, especially COPD and heart failure.

Assessment should include a full history and examination, with particular attention to past experience of flying. If possible, assess oxygen saturation levels using a finger pulse oximeter: if the value is above 95%, there should be no problem; if less than 92%, there is considerable risk of severe hypoxia from the reduced cabin pressure (and therefore inspiratory oxygen levels) present in commercial aircraft. Levels of 92–95% should prompt referral of the patient to a chest physician for vitalograph measurements and, if available, a trial of air containing 16% oxygen and assessing subsequent arterial oxygen saturations.

Patients with severe asthma should be advised against high-altitude destinations such as Nepal, Bogota, La Paz, Quito and Tibet.

■ Patients with severe asthma should be advised to carry their inhalers in their hand luggage (many are put off by the airlines' advice not to carry aerosols on the aircraft).

■ Large-volume spacers should be used rather than nebulizers (*see Q. 4.140–Q. 4.143*). If nebulizers must be used, the patient should inform the airline well in advance.

■ Many airlines will provide supplemental oxygen during flights for emergency use, often at extra cost.

■ If a patient has severe or unstable asthma, and wishes to travel on an aeroplane, they should be assessed by their general practitioner, referred if appropriate to a chest specialist, and – most importantly – contact the medical department of the airline with which they propose to travel for advice and guidance, well in advance of the proposed travel dates.

PRIMARY PREVENTION OF ASTHMA

5.96   Can asthma be prevented?

There is no proven preventive therapy. There are no strategies yet identified that might reduce the risk of atopic diseases in the population as a whole. Efforts have been focused on identifying and removing or eliminating the major environmental allergens, especially in individuals at high risk of atopy. No study has, to date, been very successful with this strategy.

Attempts have been made to identify newborn infants at risk of developing asthma by measuring cord immunoglobulin (Ig)E levels: the higher the level, the more likely is the child to develop asthma in later life. Older children may have high total IgE levels and positive radioallergosorbent test (RAST) results to house dust mite, cat dander or grass pollen, all of which are associated with increased risk of later developing atopic asthma. The manifestation of one form of atopic disease is a risk factor for the manifestation of other forms. Atopic dermatitis often occurs in the first 3 months of life and is strongly associated with the later development of atopic asthma. There is some evidence that treatment for 18 months with an oral antihistamine may at least delay, if not prevent, the onset of asthma in children identified as being at high risk of developing asthma, as detailed above.

5.97 What advice can we give to a prospective mother worried that her children may develop asthma?

An infant who prefers not to develop asthma should choose:

- Non-atopic parents
- To be a girl
- To have a mother who does not smoke in pregnancy but who does breast-feed
- A mother who avoids house dust mites, cats, pollens and other common allergens during her pregnancy
- A household where no one smokes
- Not to be born prematurely
- Not to be born in the spring
- To be part of a large family, and preferably not be the eldest
- To be brought up in an environment that is not too clean and sterile.

5.98 Can environmental changes reduce the risks of developing asthma?

There is no firm evidence for this. However, a study from the USA[15] looked at whether changes in air quality caused by relocation were associated with changes in lung function growth rates in children aged 10–15 years. The study showed that subjects who moved to areas with low levels of particulate pollution had increased rates of growth in lung function, and those who moved to areas of high pollution had lower rates. This finding may have implications for the development of COPD in later life, and may or may not be relevant for assessing the risks of developing asthma.

REFRACTIVE ASTHMA

5.99 **What do I do with the asthmatic who is not getting better despite all my efforts?**

Consider the following questions.

Is the diagnosis right?

It is always a good idea to revise the criteria on which the patient's asthma was diagnosed. Take a careful history and examine the patient for signs of other illnesses, especially heart disease. If there is diagnostic doubt, get a second opinion from a specialist. The diagnosis is hardest to make in babies and the elderly.

One of the pitfalls is the failure to establish reversibility of the patient's airway obstruction. Patients with no or little reversibility have COPD rather than asthma and should be treated as such, using the guidelines specific for the management of COPD rather than those of asthma.[12]

Is the patient taking the right drugs? Is the asthma not getting better merely because it is undertreated?

This is probably the commonest reason in practice. Take a careful history, being sure to elucidate all the patient's symptoms. As importantly, is the patient actually taking the drugs? Assessing compliance is difficult (*see Q. 5.74–Q. 5.78*). Asking patients to bring all their medication to appointments will at least allow a full assessment of how much has been taken, and this can be compared with the clinician's estimate of how much should have been taken. Enquiring as to which prescriptions have actually been dispensed can also be informative. Ask patients what they are actually taking, not what they should be taking. Ask, too, how often they forget to take each drug (this approach acknowledges that perfect compliance is not unusual and is often very difficult).

Is the patient inhaling the drugs correctly?

Always check inhaler technique in a patient who is deteriorating or not improving. No treatment works unless it is taken correctly.

Is the patient avoiding triggers correctly?

Occasionally patients will continue to be exposed to potent triggers of their asthma and be insufficiently treated to prevent the triggers from exacerbating the symptoms. This may be especially true for occupational asthma. A careful history of potential triggers should be taken and the appropriate, individualized advice given in each case. If there is persistent exposure to a trigger that cannot or will not be reduced, the preventive medication needs to be increased.

Does the patient have a reason not to get better?

Some patients may have much to gain by remaining unwell. The asthma may be their reason for avoiding occupations, relationships, duties or lifestyles that they consciously or subconsciously reject. There may be financial gain from asthma. Poorer families receiving a disabled living allowance, paid to parents who need to give care above that of usual parenting, may have a huge financial disincentive from improving their child's asthma. Compliance is likely to be particularly poor in such circumstances.

Has the patient seen the right person?

If the patient is not getting better despite a review of the diagnosis, the drugs, the regimen, the device technique, compliance and trigger avoidance, it is often worthwhile asking a colleague to review the patient and management. This can be another general practitioner or a nurse from within your primary healthcare team or, if available, a GPSI (GP with a Special Interest). Usually, hospital referral is recommended. Remember, many patients may have psychological problems that prevent them getting better. Other patients may have a subconscious motive for not getting better. However, don't be ready to accept the reasons for a patient's worsening asthma or failure to improve without careful assessment of all the other possible reasons listed above.

Is the patient anxious?

Asthma is common. Chronic anxiety is common. Some patients have both conditions. The theoretical management of the patient's asthma may be perfect, but unless the patient's underlying anxiety and its manifestations of hyperventilation (either chronic or episodic) are addressed control of the asthma will be poor. Anxious people are more accurate in their perception of airway obstruction than non-anxious people. Such people are not only more sensitive to small changes of airway obstruction, but often respond by hyperventilating, which in turn worsens the dyspnoea and distress. Usually such patients' symptoms are more severe than objective measurements of their airway obstruction. Patients are then often labelled as hysterical or overreacting, so worsening their overt dyspnoea and distress and long-term anxiety traits. This pattern is seen at its most extreme in patients with type 1 brittle asthma. The cycle can, however, be broken by careful assessment and the correct diagnosis of asthma *and* anxiety. A holistic approach involving psychotherapy assessment and teaching deep breathing and control-of-breathing exercises can be very rewarding for patients and carers.

In general, the most common reasons for a patient with asthma not getting better despite receiving the appropriate treatment are:
■ Poor inhaler technique
■ Poor compliance with treatment
■ The wrong diagnosis.

5.100 What can I do about patients who frequently attend the local accident and emergency department or walk-in centre?

Asthmatic patients who make frequent attendances to A&E departments or walk-in centres are often undertreated, despite receiving regular surveillance from their general practitioner or practice nurse. It can sometimes be difficult to assess fully the reasons for the patient's frequent attendances at these places. The attendances may simply be more convenient for the patient, or the patient may not have an adequate self-management plan, or may not fully understand how to use it. Compliance with long-term medication may be poor. Simply treating the asthma in the A&E department or walk-in centre and returning the patient to their usual care results in returning them to poor control, frequent exacerbations and reuse of the department or centre. It is probably worthwhile referring such patients for a specialist assessment.

5.101 Why and when should I follow-up patients who have been seen in the hospital or walk-in centre?

Follow-up of every asthmatic after such attendance should be made by the general practitioner or practice nurse. Ideally the A&E department or walk-in centre should strongly encourage patients to visit their practice nurse or GP soon after discharge. Attendance at the A&E department or walk-in centre can be considered to some extent as a failure of that patient's previous management, and it provides the opportunity to educate and alter treatment in order to prevent further attacks. For this to be achieved there should be prompt and affective communication between hospital or walk-in centre and GP. This is actually cost-effective in that it will reduce the chances of readmission. This appointment will allow the reasons for the event to be reviewed, and to see what failings in the self-management plan occurred. The self-management plan can then be reviewed and revised. The patient may need to step up their maintenance treatment, if they haven't already. The management of the patient's acute asthma can also be reviewed, and any deficiencies in the provision of care can be highlighted and hopefully not repeated. Relevant changes in the practice's asthma protocols can be made.

GUIDELINES AND PROTOCOLS

5.102 When were asthma guidelines introduced in the UK?

Before the late 1980s, asthma management in primary care was very informal and *ad hoc*. The quality of management depended largely on the enthusiasm of the clinicians involved.

The British Thoracic Society (BTS) published the first national guidelines, which were used not only in the UK but also in many other countries, in 1990.[16] The first American guidelines[17] were produced in 1992, as were the first international management guidelines.[18] The publication and distribution of the 1993 BTS revised guidelines[19] greatly increased the consensus amongst all clinicians. Their introduction was one of several influences that led to the continuing improvement in asthma care in the UK and in many other countries. The guidelines were last revised in 2003[22] (www.sign.ac.uk/guidelines).

All of these guidelines have helped put together the consensus on the management of asthma in adults and children. The publication and distribution of the 1993 guidelines was one of the most important influences on the evolution of modern asthma management in primary care in the UK. A survey undertaken in British general practice in 1996[20] showed that 95% of GPs were aware of the guidelines and the vast majority had changed how they managed asthma as a result of them. Moreover, their practice nurses were also aware of the guidelines and followed the advice given in them.

5.103 Why do we need the latest BTS/SIGN guidelines?

The BTS guidelines were updated in 1997[21] and reflected changes in knowledge and – as importantly – implementation of care as practised in both primary and secondary care. The BTS/SIGN guidelines[22] of 2003 again updated the guidelines and reflected best practice. The BTS/SIGN guidelines are meticulously evidence-based rather than purely consensus-based, which should encourage their use even further than the previous ones.

The new guidelines also conform more to the Global Initiatives for Asthma (GINA) guidelines[23] (used extensively in North America and much of Europe).

5.104 What is new in the 2003 BTS/SIGN asthma guidelines?

Comparing them to the 1995 BTS guidelines, the main changes are:[22]

■ The 2003 guidelines are evidence-based.

■ The emphasis is now on starting nearly all asthmatics on 'an appropriate dose' of inhaled steroids. This dose will remain fixed for most asthmatics. Fluctuations in control will be managed by the addition of other therapies, or by altering the dosage.

■ Inhaled long-acting β_2-agonists are the first-choice medication at Step 3.

■ The option of high-dose inhaled steroids is now reserved for patients with more severe asthma (Step 4) whose disease is not controlled by low-to-moderate doses of inhaled steroids with inhaled long-acting β_2-agonists.

■ Most other therapeutic options are in Step 4 (LRTAs, theophyllines, anticholinergics, cromogens, oral long-acting β_2-agonists).

■ There will be more patients at Steps 3 and 4 and fewer at Step 2 than there would be following the advice of the 1995 BTS guidelines.

5.105 Why do some organizations have their own guidelines as well?

Many practices have also adapted the BTS guidelines for their own use, as have many health trusts and authorities, and primary care trusts. Such adoptions lead to the introduction of local guidelines that are adaptations of national guidelines, specific to the need of the local population or to the local organization of care. They may lead to even greater compliance with those guidelines by all those providing asthma care. Local guidelines should be drawn up by all interested parties, including local GPs, practice and community nurses, school nurses, pharmacists, hospital paediatricians, chest physicians, geriatricians, and A&E doctors and nurses. Local guidelines should ideally be a simplification or clarification of existing guidelines, and should aim to produce consistent standards of care in any particular locality.

5.106 What is the difference between a guideline and a protocol?

Guidelines are proposals based on consensus and evidence that are deliberately non-directive. They make no attempt to suggest how the advice given in them should be implemented. They are a means of advising those who provide asthma care on the essential points of that care.

Asthma protocols are agreements drawn up by organizations directly involved in providing asthma care, specifying how that care will be delivered and how the advice given in guidelines will be implemented. It is essentially a primary care trust's or practice's way of agreeing what it will do and how it will do it.

5.107 What should a practice protocol for asthma contain?

The following should be agreed.

DIAGNOSIS

■ Diagnostic criteria
■ Use of peak flow diaries and trials of treatment
■ Responsibility for making and recording the diagnosis and sharing it with the patient or carer.

MANAGEMENT

■ Aims of management
■ Who will give the relevant advice, education and follow-up
■ Trigger avoidance, including smoking
■ Treatment, including choice of drugs and delivery systems, peak flow meters, self-management or action plans, follow-up after any exacerbation
■ Audit and quality control.

REFERRALS

■ Criteria for referral to secondary care or from nurse to GP, and vice versa
■ Criteria for referral to other healthcare professionals and agencies.

5.108 How often should we review well patients?

All asthmatic patients should be reviewed at least annually. The following groups of patients should be reviewed more frequently:

■ *Children*: babies as often as monthly, preschool-aged children 3–6 monthly, school-aged children at least every six months.
■ *Elderly or patients with co-morbidity*: every 3–6 months.
■ *Pregnant women*: at every antenatal appointment.
■ *Those who needed emergency attention* in the previous six months (night visit, A& E or walk-in centre attendance): as soon as possible after the event, then 1–2 monthly until stable.
■ *Those who needed admission* with a severe exacerbation of asthma: as soon as possible after the event, then every month for at least six months.

5.109 Who should review the patients?

This will depend on the skills mix and experience of the doctors and nurses in the practice. In most UK practices there is at least one nurse who has received specialist asthma training and has experience in managing asthma.

It seems sensible for this nurse to review the majority of the asthmatics, especially those who are well controlled at Steps 1–3. Patients with poorly controlled asthma or more severe asthma should be managed by more experienced nurses, or by the GP. All patients should be offered the option of whom they see, if practicable.

5.110 What should we do at the review appointment?

At each review the clinician should:

- Make a detailed enquiry of symptoms and lifestyle impairment
- Check (and adjust if necessary) the inhaler technique
- Check compliance with management
- Check peak flow readings and charts, if relevant
- Educate, listen and explain
- Check the self-management plan. Does the patient know how and when to recognize deterioration; how and when to alter treatment; and how and when to call for help?

AUDIT

5.111 What is audit?

Audit is nothing more than looking at what one is doing and comparing it with what one would like to be doing, and trying to make the two identical.

5.112 Why audit asthma care?

Asthma is well suited to general practice audit because it is common and there are recognized, measurable outcomes and processes. Asthma audit should involve the team that is involved in asthma care, and not be the responsibility of only one member. It is only by looking at what we are doing that we can assess whether we are doing it correctly. Practices that have audited outcomes of their asthma care have found that the audits can help to bring about measurable improvements in the quality of care that is delivered to asthmatic patients.

5.113 What are the principles behind auditing my asthma care?

The cardinal rules of all audit are to keep it simple, to keep it specific, and to keep it relevant. As a practice's experience grows, audit can move from the very simple to the more complex. There are three parts to a successful asthma audit:

1 *Measures of fact*: e.g. practice prevalence of asthma, clinic attendance.
2 *Measures of process*: e.g. how many asthmatics own a peak flow meter? How many have had a peak flow measurement recorded in the last year?

How many are on inhaled steroids or anti-inflammatories, or other measure of appropriate treatment?

3 *Measures of outcome*: e.g. how many home visits or emergency admissions there were per month, daily/nocturnal symptom scores, inhaler technique ability, compliance with medication, time off work or school.

The most valuable information lies in measuring outcomes. Processes are only ways of achieving the outcomes, not ends in themselves.

5.114 What do I need to audit?

To claim chronic disease management payments for asthma in the UK, each practice is required to provide the health authority with the following information:

■ The number of patients with asthma
■ The percentage of asthmatics receiving prophylactic therapy
■ The percentage who have had a peak flow measurement recorded in the last 12 months
■ The number of asthmatic patients who have received a statutory review of their asthma in last 12 months.

All of these requirements are process measures and do not really provide an objective assessment of the quality of asthma care. The practice should concentrate more on auditing outcome, especially hospital admissions.

5.115 What do I do with my audit results?

Audit is basically a cycle. The results of the initial audit should be used to test practice procedures so that the standards of asthma care that have been agreed will be met. If the initial standards are too low (i.e. easily met) or too high (not nearly met), the standards may need raising or lowering. The audit cycle is shown in *Fig. 5.1*.

5.116 What should I audit?

Each practice must decide which areas of asthma management to audit; the practice must also set criteria and agreed standards. Some examples include:

■ *Measures of fact*: to establish the practice prevalence rate for adults and children, and to compare this with national rates; to see every asthmatic at least annually. It is important to try to maintain a dynamic asthma register. This is one that allows patients who have gone into remission and who remained in remission for a specified length of time to be removed from the register, as well as the ability to add new patients once they are diagnosed.

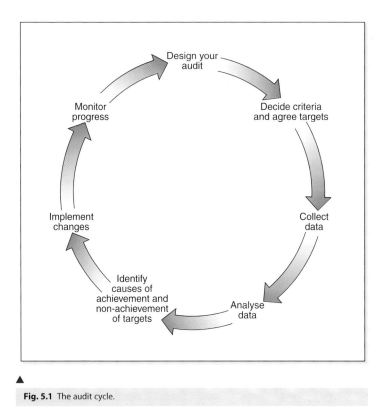

Fig. 5.1 The audit cycle.

- *Measures of process*: to achieve a 50% rate of asthmatics owning a peak flow meter; to have recorded a peak flow reading in the last year for all asthmatics aged 5 years or more; to have 100% of asthmatics who require more than four relieving inhalers a year to be using preventive inhalers regularly as well.
- *Measure of outcome*: to achieve no hospital admissions due to acute asthma, no emergency nebulizations and no home visits; 100% of asthmatics with *good* inhaler technique and no asthmatics suffering nocturnal symptoms.

5.117 How do I collect the data?

In the UK, most data are collected from computer records and are therefore reliant on the clinician accurately recording the data at the time of each consultation or review. Data retrieval depends on data input. It is often necessary to review the asthma protocol and to insert or delete the need to record certain data. Adequate data recording is essential for all audit, but it is often not until audit is undertaken that deficiencies of data input become apparent.

5.118 What do I do with these data?

The data need to be analysed. The results achieved should be compared with the standards set. Discrepancies should be highlighted and attempts made to identify the causes of any non-achievement. For example, if the practice has an adult prevalence rate of 14% and a childhood prevalence of 6% compared with national estimates of 5% and 10% respectively, why is this? Are the diagnostic standards inappropriately wide for adults and too narrow for children? Similarly, low ownership of peak flow meters may be due to lack of awareness on the part of the professional carers about how useful they can be. The subject may have been omitted from the clinic protocols. Failure to meet the outcome standards may be due to faulty clinical protocols, inadequate monitoring, training or education, or inappropriate prescribing, poor use of self-management plans or inappropriate advice – or any combination.

5.119 How do I know what changes to make?

Having identified the causes of non-achievement of standards, changes should be implemented so that they can be achieved. Unrealistic standards may need to be modified. If the standard was appropriate but unmet, changes in the provision of care must be made. If attendance at the asthma clinic is low, is this because it is held at an inconvenient time or place? Is failure to review every asthmatic annually due to inadequate provision of clinic time or to poor organization, so that not all patients are called and recalled? If too few asthmatics are using preventive treatment, is this because the treatment protocols are wrong, or is the training of those running the clinic inadequate, or is the advice not being complied with by patients? If outcome measures fall short of the standards, is this due to poor care, to good care that is badly organized, or do the practice's asthmatics have dreadful asthma despite excellent care and management?

5.120 How do I make the necessary changes?

The final stage is to implement changes to protocols, procedures, standards and provision of care, and then to re-evaluate, monitor progress and re-audit. It is only by looking critically at the effects of change that we can evaluate that change. Not all change is necessarily good.

Having agreed with the practice the reasons for not achieving some of the standards that you have set, the practice needs to develop an action plan to remedy these specific areas. For example, it may be useful to promote a protocol that any patient who has needed an emergency nebulization should also receive oral steroids, have their peak flow measured before and after the nebulization, be reviewed in an asthma clinic within a specified time after the event, and have a self-management plan initiated or reviewed. The practice can then look at how patients who received emergency nebulizations were managed in subsequent years and see whether there have been improvements.

5.121 Isn't audit a bit boring and depressing?

Audit can be uplifting, interesting or sometimes dispiriting. It is better to keep audit very simple and to confine oneself to asking simple questions that involve easy data collection and analysis, and that have fairly straightforward causes of non-achievement, and where it is easy to make small, beneficial changes. At first it is also best to audit simple aspects of asthma care where it is believed that the practice is doing well, to provide positive feedback for the whole team. As confidence increases, so can the complexity of audits: there can be more concentration on the aspects that are probably being done less well and are therefore in greater need of change. A more experienced, confident team can cope with negative feedback.

5.122 Does audit show that asthma clinics make any difference to the provision of asthma care?

The answer is probably that they do, but whether the improvement comes from having nurse-run asthma clinics or from the practice developing an interest in asthma, with protocols, self-management plans and peak flow meter use is difficult to know. It is more certain that patient education alone is insufficient to alter morbidity. A review of audits, facilitators and childhood asthma has been undertaken in Scotland.[24] The intervention group had a fall in the number of hospital inpatient days compared with quite a large rise in the control group. What is more, the total healthcare costs of the control group rose during the year studied by a much greater extent than the cost for the intervention group.

5.123 What about more sophisticated audits?

More sophisticated audits may be more difficult to carry out, partly because of difficulties in data collection and analysis. Most general practice computer systems are better at collecting data that involve either the absence or presence of something, than at determining the number of those things. Most of the systems currently in use are not useful for gathering information on, for instance, the number of prescriptions the patient may have received of a particular drug over a particular timespan or, as another example, the number of days lost from work due to asthma.

More sophisticated measures of morbidity could include:

- *Nocturnal and early morning symptoms* – these are common manifestations of poor asthma control.
- *Daytime and activity-induced symptoms* – patients are often reluctant to acknowledge this limitation. Asking patients whether normal daily activities bring on symptoms is one way of addressing daytime symptoms.
- *Days lost to asthma* – this is a measure of morbidity as this reflects the impact of asthma on the patient's lifestyle. These data are very subjective, and patients are notoriously inaccurate in remembering the number of days that they may have lost from work or school, especially if you ask them to delve too far back into their memory.
- *Reliever use* – auditing the number of prescriptions for relieving medications over a six-month period can help to identify patients with a high asthma morbidity. On the whole, a large number of reliever prescriptions indicates poor asthma control, unless the asthma is very severe.

The following measures of patient management can also be evaluated:

- Inhaler technique – poor inhaler technique is a major cause of failure of treatment. Inhaler technique should be checked at every opportunity.
- Does each patient have their own individual guidelines or self-management plan?

Asthma in the future

6

6.1	Do we need any new drugs for asthma?	224
6.2	What new drugs might be available for asthma in the future?	224
6.3	Is there any scope for improving trigger avoidance?	225
6.4	Are there any advances in immunology that might be of clinical benefit?	226
6.5	Are there any advances in genetics that might be of clinical benefit?	226
6.6	Will asthma therapies become more specific?	227
	Summary	227

PQ PATIENT QUESTIONS

6.7	My son takes a brown puffer twice a day and a blue one when needed, via a spacer. He starts school next week. What should I do about his inhalers?	229
6.8	My granny is aged 80 and has asthma. She should take a purple inhaler twice a day and a blue one if she needs it, but she keeps forgetting and tells me they don't work even when she does take them. She is quite breathless most of the time. What should I do?	229
6.9	Will there ever be a cure for asthma?	229

6.1 Do we need any new drugs for asthma?

The existing treatments for asthma are safe and effective. However, for therapy to be fully effective, multiple drugs are often needed. There are still lingering doubts about inhaled steroids, especially in high doses, and very real and reasonable concerns regarding long-term use of oral steroids. Compliance with inhaled therapy continues to be a problem and is lower than for oral therapy. The ideal treatment is probably a once-daily tablet that completely controls asthma without any side-effects.

6.2 What new drugs might be available for asthma in the future?

New bronchodilators

A long-acting anticholinergic agent called tiotropium has been developed which is taken once daily. This is probably going to be more useful in the management of chronic obstructive pulmonary disease (COPD) than in asthma. Revatropate is an oral anticholinergic drug that is currently being evaluated. Potassium channel openers have been advocated for use in asthma but they have proven to be fairly ineffective and their use is limited by side-effects. Vasoactive inhibitory peptide (VIP) is a potent bronchodilator, but unfortunately the dosage needed to produce bronchodilatation results in massive vasodilatation, and is therefore only really suitable for people who are permanently lying down. Inhaled indomethacin has been shown to reduce the fall in the forced expiratory volume in 1 second (FEV_1) following exercise in children with exercise-induced asthma. Nebulized magnesium sulfate has been shown to have a significant bronchodilator effect in acute asthma but its use in clinical practice is uncertain.

New inhaled steroids

New developments currently being researched are depot inhaled steroids, which will need to be taken only once a day or perhaps even less frequently. New steroids, such as ciclesonide, are also being researched that may have an increased topical affect on the airways with even fewer systemic effects than those currently on the market. Steroids that work at a more specific biochemical level of the inflammatory process are also being investigated. Triamcinolone is licensed as an inhaled steroid in the USA but seems to be no better than the existing steroids licensed in the UK (beclometasone, budesonide, fluticasone and mometasone).

Immunomodulatory treatment

Neither methotrexate nor ciclosporin has been widely accepted as a useful drug in the long-term management of severe asthma.

A cytokine inhibitor called mycohenolat, which can be given as an intravenous bolus injection, has some immunomodulatory effect, which can last for up to three months. Much attention has been paid to prostaglandin E, which is a potent bronchodilator but is ineffective if given by inhalation.

Phosphodiesterases are chemicals involved in the inflammatory response. There are many different types of phosphodiesterase, and therefore many different types of inhibitor. At present none seems to have much clinical use, but it may be that more specific phosphodiesterase inhibitors will be developed in the near future. Some phosphodiesterase inhibitors appeared to have anti-inflammatory and bronchodilator effects in animal studies and in some early human studies.

Anti-immunoglobulin E therapy

Novel immunological treatments for asthma have been proposed in recent attempts to improve IgE-mediated allergic reactions and to reduce the severity of asthma. Several randomized, double-blind, parallel, placebo-controlled studies have examined the effects of the anti-IgE agent omalizumab, injected intravenously in adult and childhood asthma.[1] Exacerbation rates and steroid use both declined by up to 50% and markers of the early and the late phase inflammatory response were attenuated significantly. This represents a breakthrough in the concepts of asthma therapy, and omalizumab may be useful in patients with severe symptoms or with multiple allergies. Omalizumab needs to be given by injection, probably weekly, and is likely to be expensive.

Chloride channel blockers

Inhaled furosemide (frusemide) has been used and provides potent bronchodilatation, but unfortunately this effect lasts for only about an hour.

6.3   Is there any scope for improving trigger avoidance?

Much work has been done on allergen avoidance. The next step would appear to be to use the recent advances in our knowledge and understanding of allergies to provide personal advice on allergen avoidance as well as community advice. It is also becoming increasingly apparent that targeting allergen avoidance intervention at an early stage of life may be beneficial. Certainly, reducing the allergen load on newborn infants who have a strong family history of atopy or allergies has resulted in reductions in such children's immune response to common allergens. The next stage is to see whether avoidance of allergens by pregnant women, together with avoidance of allergens by babies in the first year of life, will be even more beneficial. Studies are currently taking place to evaluate this hypothesis.

6.4 Are there any advances in immunology that might be of clinical benefit?

The structure of the allergenic protein produced by the house dust mite has been determined. The next challenge is to modify the protein so that its structure is maintained but its enzyme acitivty is lost. This inactivated form of protein could form the basis of a vaccine for people who are sensitive to the house dust mite.

Recent advances in molecular biological techniques have allowed greater understanding of the precise mechanisms involved in allergic asthma. As part of that immune response, large quantities of IgE antibodies are produced which attach to mast cells and release histamine and other mediators. It is these mediators that cause acute symptoms of asthma. If the overproduction of IgE could be controlled, asthma and other allergic diseases might also be controlled. There is a cluster of genes on chromosome 5 that produce interleukins that stimulate the production of IgE. If either the genes could be switched off or the interleukins antagonized or blocked, it might be possible to control allergic asthma. However, there are other chemical substances involved in the immune response, including tumour necrosis factor (TNF) and T-helper lymphocytes. If the TNF or T helper cells could be 'switched off' in the first few years of life when allergy first develops, this might prevent susceptible children from developing allergic asthma. As the precise chemicals in allergic responses are identified, so are the genes that control them, and it may be possible to generate specific and selective treatments that will block the processes that lead to the development of asthma.

6.5 Are there any advances in genetics that might be of clinical benefit?

There are probably multiple genes linked to the development of asthma; some involve atopy and others influence airway responsiveness. However, the ability to identify genes that are important to the development of asthma has a number of practical consequences. If a gene variant could be identified that markedly altered airway activity, for example, it might be possible to use gene therapy strategies to negate the influence of that genetic variant. This is unlikely to be a practical, viable treatment option, except perhaps for some highly selected patients with severe disease unresponsive to other therapies. There are obvious ethical considerations to gene therapy, and cheaper and effective pharmacological agents are available that adequately control the vast majority of patients.

ADAM33, a gene associated with airway remodelling, has recently been identified. Further work may allow the development of therapies targeted at this gene and its products, to prevent the onset of airway remodelling. Currently all asthmatics are treated with long-term inhaled steroids in order to reduce the risk of a proportion of them developing airway remodelling; as we are unable to identify which patients comprise that proportion, all patients are managed this way even though only a minority will benefit. Eventually it may be possible to screen infants to identify those at risk of asthma, and then to prevent the gene from being switched on.

6.6   Will asthma therapies become more specific?

Asthma may be seen as a syndrome that encompasses a variety of pathologies, symptom complexes and disorders of the airways. We may in future view the disease as 'Asthmas', and be able to differentiate the various types more easily and more accurately. It may well be that only certain children with symptoms attributable to asthma will actually have chronic airway inflammation. The remainder of such children will become less troubled by their symptoms as they grow older. Those who do have chronic airway inflammation, and the adults who develop it *de novo*, may be further subdivided into those who will develop airway remodelling and those who will not. Finally, only some of the patients at risk of airway remodelling will develop it, because effective long-term treatment with inhaled steroids over the years will have prevented the development of airway remodelling. At present we do not know which asthmatics are most at risk of developing airway remodelling, which can lead to worsening asthma and the development of irreversible airways obstruction. We tend, therefore, to treat all patients with long-term preventive therapy, whereas it may be the case that only certain groups of patients will benefit. The problem at present is that we do not know which patients will derive most benefit.

SUMMARY

Asthma is a complex and common disease affecting people of all ages, and which can start at any age. Despite much being known about its pathogenesis, no cure is currently feasible. Asthma is still a common cause of disability, illness and sometimes death.

By applying and combining all that is known about successful asthma management, general practice teams should be able to provide good standards of care for their asthmatic patients. This should lead to less illness and disability, and to improvements in the quality of life for nearly all asthmatics. The platforms of good asthma care are:

■ Patient and clinician education
■ Proper use of the sophisticated drug treatments, delivery devices and regimens
■ The organization of shared proactive care by general practice teams together with their patients.

Asthma is a common disease but need not be a common reason for underachievement, failure to fulfil potential, illness or disability. Good asthma care is effective, easily achievable by primary care teams, and very rewarding.

PQ PATIENT QUESTIONS

6.7 My son takes a brown puffer twice a day and a blue one when needed, via a spacer. He starts school next week. What should I do about his inhalers?

The problem really concerns the use of his reliever inhaler: who decides when he needs it and who helps him to use it? It is realistic to allow all children some say as to when they think they need their reliever inhaler, and you and your son should talk about this matter and agree the criteria, using language he understands. He should be encouraged to use his spacer with minimal supervision. You will need to talk to your son's teacher and let the teacher know about your son's asthma, and when he is likely to need to use his reliever. Children aged 5 years are probably too young to be in complete control of their medication at school (although most can do this by age 7 or 8), so the teacher will need to be in charge of the storage and use of the inhaler and spacer. Most schools have an Asthma Policy. If your son's school does not, ask them to obtain a school pack from the National Asthma Campaign (http://www.asthma.org.uk; 0345 010203). You should also talk to the school nurse about your son and his asthma management.

6.8 My granny is aged 80 and has asthma. She should take a purple inhaler twice a day and a blue one if she needs it, but she keeps forgetting and tells me they don't work even when she does take them. She is quite breathless most of the time. What should I do?

There are several issues here:

- Is the diagnosis right? In the elderly, the most common diagnoses that can be confused with asthma are COPD or heart failure. Is your granny on other tablets, and does she take them as she should? If she hasn't seen her doctor recently, why don't you go with her to see the doctor and explain your concerns?
- Is she using the inhalers correctly? Poor inhaler technique means that the drugs will not work properly. Is the inhaler technique hampered by poor memory, poor eyesight, tremor or arthritis of the hands? If so, a different device may help – again, ask your granny to see her doctor or nurse.
- Is her forgetfulness more than occasional memory loss? If you or your granny is worried about this, visit her doctor together.

6.9 Will there ever be a cure for asthma?

Certainly, no cure is likely within the next few years. Asthma is a very complex disease caused by a mixture of genetic and environmental factors that interact to variable extents between individuals and even in the same individual at different times. In other words, a cure is unlikely because there is not just one – or even a few – easily identifiable causes or effects.

Generic name	Brand name	MDI	Inhalers — Compatible spacer	Inhalers — Breath-actuated inhaler or DPD	Other preparations
1. β₂-Agonists (short acting)					
Salbutamol	Aerolin			Autohaler	
	Airomir	✓	Aerochamber	Autohaler	
	Asmasal		Clickhaler		
	Salbutamol		Pulvinal	Novolizer	
	Salamol	✓		Easi-Breathe	
	Salbulin	✓	Aerochamber		
	Salbutamol Ventodisks			Ventodisks	
	Ventolin	✓	Volumatic Babyhaler	Accuhaler	Syrup
	Ventolin Evo-haler	✓	Volumatic Babyhaler		
	Volmax				Tablets
Terbutaline	Bricanyl	✓	Nebuhaler	Turbohaler	Tablets or syrup
Orciprenaline	Alupent				Tablets or syrup
2. Corticosteroids (inhaled)					
Beclometasone	Aerobec			Autohaler	
	Aerobec Forte			Autohaler	
	Asmabec	✓		Clickhaler	
	Beclazone			Easi-Breathe	
	Becloforte	✓	Volumatic	Diskhaler	
	Beclometasone			Pulvinal	
	Becodisks			Becodisks	
	Becotide	✓	Volumatic Babyhaler		

Generic name	Brand name	Inhalers MDI	Compatible spacer	Breath-actuated inhaler or DPD	Other preparations
	Filair Forte	✓			
	Filair	✓			
	Qvar	✓	Aerochamber	Autohaler Novolizer Turbohaler	
Budesonide	Pulmicort	✓	Nebuhaler NebuChamber		
Fluticasone	Flixotide	✓	Volumatic	Disks Accuhaler	
Mometasone	Asmanex			Twisthaler	
Prednisolone					Tablets Soluble tablets
3. Non-steroidal anti-inflammatory drugs					
Cromoglicate	Intal	✓	Fisonair Syncroner	Easi-Breathe	Spincaps
Nedocromil	Tilade	✓	Syncroner		
Ketotifen	Zaditen				Tablets
4. β_2-Agonists (long acting)					
Bambuterol	Bambec				Tablets
Formoterol (eformoterol)	Foradil			Aerolizer Turbohaler	
	Oxis				
Salmeterol	Serevent	✓	Volumatic	Disks Accuhaler	

Generic name	Brand name	MDI	Inhalers Compatible spacer	Breath-actuated inhaler or DPD	Other preparations
5. Anticholinergic drugs					
Ipratropium	Atrovent	✓		Aerocaps Autohaler	
Oxitropium	Atrovent Forte Oxivent	✓ ✓		Autohaler	
6. Combination drugs					
Cromoglicate + salbutamol	Aerocrom	✓	Syncroner		
Fenoterol + ipratropium	Duovent	✓		Autohaler	
Salbutamol + ipratropium	Combivent	✓			
Salmeterol + fluticasone	Seretide	✓	Volumatic	Accuhaler	
Budenoside + formoterol (eformoterol)	Symbicort			Easi-Breathe Turbohaler	
TABLETS					
7. Leukotriene antagonists					
Montelukast	Singulair				
Zafirlukast	Accolate				

Generic name	Brand name	Inhalers			Other preparations
		MDI	Compatible spacer	Breath-actuated inhaler or DPD	
8. *Theophyllines*					
Aminophylline	Not branded				
Aminophylline	Phyllocontin Continus				
	Phyllocontin Paediatric				
Choline	Nuelin				
Theophylline	Slo-Phyllin				
	Theo-Dur				
	Uniphyllin Continus				

DPD, dry powder device; MDI, metered-dose inhaler

APPENDIX B
Devices and drugs currently available in the UK: manufacturers' designs

DEVICE		DRUG		
Brand name	Type	Generic name	Brand name	Dosages available (µg per dose)
Accuhaler	DP	Fluticasone	Flixotide	50, 100, 250, 500
		Salbutamol	Ventolin	200
		Salmeterol	Serevent	50
		Salmeterol + fluticasone	Seretide	50–100, 50–250, 50–500
Aerohaler and Aerocaps	DP	Ipratropium	Atrovent	40
Aerolizer	DP	Formoterol (eformoterol)	Foradil	12 mg
Autohaler	BAD	Beclometasone	Aerobec and Aerobec Forte	50, 100 and 250
			Qvar	50, 100, 250
		Ipratropium	Atrovent and Atrovent Forte	20 and 40
		Ipratropium + fenoterol	Duovent	40–100
		Oxitropium	Oxivent	100
		Salbutamol	Aerolin	100
			Aerimir	100
Babyhaler	MVS	Salbutamol	Ventolin	200
		Beclometasone	Becotide 50	50
Clickhaler	DP	Salbutamol	Asmasal	95
		Beclometasone	Asmabec	50, 100, 250
Diskhaler	DP	Beclometasone	Becotide and Becloforte	100, 200, 400 and 400
		Fluticasone	Flixotide	50, 100, 250, 500
		Salbutamol	Ventolin	200, 400
		Salmeterol	Serevent	50
Easi-Breathe	BAD	Beclometasone	Beclazone	50, 100
		Salbutamol	Salamol	100
		Cromoglicate	Cromogen	5 mg

DEVICE		DRUG		
Brand name	**Type**	**Generic name**	**Brand name**	**Dosages available (μg per dose)**
Fisonair	LVS	Cromoglicate	Intal	5 mg
NebuChamber	MVS	Budesonide	Pulmicort	200
Nebuhaler	LVS	Budesonide	Pulmicort	100, 200, 400
		Terbutaline	Bricanyl	250
Novolizer	DP	Budesonide		100, 200
		Salbutamol		100
Pulvinal	DP	Beclometasone		100
		Salbutamol		200
Spacehaler	SVS	Salbutamol	Salbutamol Spacehaler	100
		Beclometasone	BDP Spacehaler	50, 100, 250
Spacer Inhaler	SVS	Budesonide	Pulmicort	100, 200, 400
		Terbutaline	Bricanyl	250
Spinhaler and Spincaps	DP	Cromoglicate	Intal	20 mg
Syncroner	SVS	Cromoglicate	Intal	5 mg
		Nedocromil	Tilade	2 mg
		Salbutamol + cromoglicate	Aerocrom	100–1000
Turbohaler	DP	Budesonide	Pulmicort	100, 200, 400
		Formoterol (eformoterol)	Oxis	6, 12
		Terbutaline	Bricanyl	500
Twisthaler	DP	Mometasone	Asmanex	200, 400
Volumatic	LVS	Beclometasone	Becotide and Becloforte	50, 100, 200 and 250
		Fluticasone	Flixotide	25, 50, 125, 250
		Salbutamol	Ventolin	100
		Salmeterol	Serevent	50
		Salmeterol + fluticasone	Seretide	50–100, 50–250, 50–500

Universal spacers for use with any MDI: Able Spacer, AeroChamber, AeroChamber Plus (all MVS)
BAD, breath-actuated device; DP, dry powder device; LVS, large-volume spacer; MVS, medium-volume spacer; SVS, small-volume spacer

APPENDIX C
Drugs currently available in the UK that are available as metered-dose inhalers

Generic name	Brand name	Dose (μg per puff)	Notes
Salbutamol + cromoglicate	Aerocrom	100–1000	
Salbutamol	Aeromir	100	CFC free
Ipratropium	Atrovent	20	
Beclometasone	Beclazone	50, 100, 250	
Beclometasone	Becloforte	250	
Beclometasone	Becotide	50, 100, 200	
Beclometasone	Qvar	50, 100	CFC free
Terbutaline	Bricanyl	250	
Salbutamol + ipratropium	Combivent	100–200	
Cromoglicate	Cromogen	5 mg	
Fenoterol + ipratropium	Duovent	40–100	
Beclometasone	Filair	50, 100, 250	
Fluticasone	Flixotide	25, 50, 125, 250	
Cromoglicate	Intal	5 mg	
Oxitropium	Oxivent	100	
Budesonide	Pulmicort	50, 200	
Salbutamol	Salamol	100	
Salbutamol	Salbulin	100	
Salmeterol + fluticasone	Seretide	25–50, 25–125, 25–250	
Salmeterol	Serevent	25	
Nedocromil	Tilade	2 mg	
Salbutamol	Ventolin Evohaler	100	CFC free

CFC, chlorofluorocarbon

APPENDIX D
Sources of information

ORGANIZATIONS

UK

The National Asthma Campaign is an effective voluntary organization that sponsors research, provides and funds professional training and support, and campaigns effectively on behalf of patients to improve the quality and quantity of care available to asthmatic patients. It produces a wide range of literature for patients.

Head office
National Asthma Campaign
Providence House
Providence Place
London N1 0NT
UK
Tel: +44 (0)20 7226 2260
Facsimile: +44 (0)20 7704 0740
Website: http://www.asthma.org.uk

National Asthma Campaign Scotland
2a North Charlotte Street
Edinburgh EH2 4HR
UK
Tel: +44 (0)131 226 2544
Facsimile: +44 (0)131 226 2401

The Asthma Helpline (Tel: 0845 7 01 02 03) is available from Monday to Friday, 9am to 7pm.

The General Practice Airways Group (GPIAG) is an independent, multifunded, general practitioner-led member organization that promotes and facilitates the highest standards of research and the best management of patients with asthma and other respiratory disorders.

GPIAG
8th Floor, Egbaston House
3 Duchess Place
Egbaston
Birmingham B16 8NH
UK

Tel: +44 (0)121 454 8219
Facsimile: +44 (0)121 454 1190
Website: http://www.gpiag.org

The National Respiratory Training Centre is a centre of excellence for the training of practice nurses (especially) and GPs in the management of asthma, allergy and respiratory disorders in primary care. Courses are available on asthma and allergy that are predominantly by distance learning, leading to a diploma.

The National Respiratory Training Centre
The Athenaeum
10 Church Street
Warwick CV34 4AB
UK
Tel: +44 (0)1926 493313
Website: http://www.nartc.org.uk

The British Lung Foundation funds research into all lung conditions, provides public information on lung diseases and good lung health, and supports people affected by lung disease through the Breathe Easy Club. The Foundation also campaigns at parliamentary and council levels of democracy for its aims. It is an excellent source of help, information and leaflets, and can offer practical advice and support to patients and primary healthcare workers.

The British Lung Foundation
National Office
78 Hatton Gardens
London EC1N 8LD
UK
Tel: +44 (0)207 831 5831
Website: http://www.lunguk.org

The **Respiratory Education and Training Centres** are based in Liverpool but run satellite courses for nurses, doctors and those in professions allied to medicine.

Respiratory Education and Training Centre
University Hospital Aintree
Lower Lane
Liverpool L9 7AL
UK
Tel: +44 (0)151 529 2598
Facsimile: +44 (0)151 529 3943
Website: http://www.respiratoryetc.com

The Lung and Asthma Information Agency provides regular and recent factsheets and data on lung conditions.

Lung and Asthma Information Agency
Department of Public Health Services
St George's Hospital Medical School
Cranmer Terrace
London SW17 0RE
Facsimile: +44 (0)208 725 3584
Website: http://www.sghms.ac.uk/depts/laia/laia.htm

Action on Smoking and Health (ASH) aims to help people to stop smoking.

Action on Smoking and Health
102 Clifton Street
London EC2A 4HW
UK
Tel: +44 (0)207 739 5902
Facsimile: +44 (0)207 613 0531
Website: http://www.ash.org.uk

QUIT is a charity that supports people who wish to stop smoking.

QUIT
Victory House
Tottenham Court Road
London WC1 0HA
UK
Tel: +44 (0)207 388 5775
Facsimile: +44 (0)207 388 5995
Quitline: 0800 002200 (for callers in England)
Smokeline: 0800 848484 (for callers in Scotland)
Northern Ireland Quitline: 01232 663281 (for callers in Northern Ireland)
Smokers' Helpline: 034545 697 500 (for callers in Wales)

Quitline is also available for speakers of the following languages:

Bengali: 0800 002244 (Monday 1pm to 9pm)
Gujarati: 0800 002255 (Tuesday 1pm to 9pm)
Hindi: 0800 002266 (Wednesday 1pm to 9pm)
Punjabi: 0800 002277 (Thursday 1pm to 9pm)
Urdu: 0800 002288 (Sunday 1pm to 9pm)
Turkish/Kurdish: 0800 002299 (Sunday 1pm to 9pm)

Worldwide

The International Primary Care Respiratory Group (IPCRG) is dedicated to improving the primary care of patients with respiratory disorders. It has its own on-line journal and organizes many international meetings, allowing exchange of ideas and research ideas and results across nations. Website: http://www.ipcrg.org

The **National Institutes of Health** (NIH) in the USA have produced excellent material for the care of asthma. Their website, http://www.nlm.nih.gov/medlineplus/asthma.html, is superb, containing all the information that most clinicians will ever need or want. The site is clear and easy to navigate, and extremely comprehensive.

The **World Health Organization** (WHO) has taken an active role in trying to improve the correct diagnosis and management of asthma. The Global Initiative for Asthma (GINA) guidelines were published jointly by the NIH and WHO. The WHO website, http://www.who.int/ncd/asthma, provides information on the World Health Organization, including guidelines, publication and news. It is easy to navigate, and informative.

Europe

The **European Respiratory Society** (ERS) is an international organization primarily for secondary care respiratory specialists, but with an increasing input from primary care. http://www.ersnet.org is a useful website for clinicians, especially academics. It contains news and recently published articles from the literature and recent international meetings, as well as articles published in the *European Respiratory Journal*.

The **European Federation of Allergy and Airways Diseases Patients' Association** (EFA) is an alliance of 36 organizations in 20 different countries across Europe, dedicated to improving asthma care and exchanging information and research. Its website, http://www.efanet.org, provides news and recent articles for healthcare professionals, including the results of surveys conducted in Europe.

USA

The site of the **Asthma and Allergy Foundation of America** provides information and sponsors research in the USA. It has a comprehensive and well-designed website, http://www.aafa.org, for patients and healthcare professionals, with a wealth of useful and well-presented information and news.

The **American College of Allergy, Asthma and Immunology** is an organization of allergists, immunologists and related healthcare professionals dedicated to quality patient care through research, advocacy, and public and professional education. Its website, http://www.allergy.mcg.edu, is glossy and well produced, and is fairly informative.

A large survey of asthma in the USA, sponsored by Smith Kline Glaxo, is shown at http://www.asthmainamerica.com; this site also contains useful information on the diagnosis and management of asthma in children and adults.

http://www.healthtalk.com/aen/index.html is a fun site for patients with audio dialogue discussing many of the main points in asthma management.

The **American Lung Association** is dedicated to improving the care of all patients with respiratory conditions through public and professional education as well as advocacy. Its website http://www.lungusa.org/asthma is a superb and comprehensive site for healthcare professionals and patients. It is well presented with good links.

Other websites
National organizations with ideals, aims and methods similar to those of the National Asthma Campaign in the UK exist in several countries and can be found at the following websites:

Canada

http://www.asthmasociety.com – slick and colourful with sufficient detail for most patients.
http://www.lung.ca/asthma – useful links and also national resources in Canada (for patients).

Australia

http://www.nationalasthma.org.au – a very good site with lots of information for patients and healthcare professionals. There is more in this site than first seems apparent, so don't be put off by first impressions.

http://www.asthmaaustralia.org.au – another good and informative site. The simple presentation and layout belies its quality. This is a site primarily for patients, but will be of some use to many healthcare professionals as well.

New Zealand

http://www.asthmanz.co.nz – an excellent site with lots of information, much of which is not immediately apparent, so be patient and persevere.

France

http://www.remcomp.com/asmanet/asmalink.html – this site is difficult to navigate. It should allow easy access to something called the 'asmanet', but this seems to be little more than a search on Google, using the words keyed in by the user. It seems more sensible to go straight to Google (http://www.google.com).

Ireland

http://www.asthmasociety.ie – a better site than first impressions may give, with lots of useful information plainly portrayed. Try to ignore the shopping baskets and supermarket-type marketing.

South Africa

http://www.asthma.co.za – a fairly comprehensive site with good information for patients.

OTHER USEFUL WEBSITES

Asthma guidelines

http://www.nhlbi.nih.gov/guidelines/asthma/asthgdln.htm – comprehensive updates of the GINA guidelines with good links to further resources. Patient and healthcare professional sections.

http://www.ginasthma.com – the original GINA with updates and links.

http://www.brit-thoracic.org.uk/sign/index.htm – the latest British guidelines on asthma management, with some background and related information.

http://www.sign.ac.uk/guidelines/published/support/guideline 63/download.html – the latest UK guidelines, now evidence based and referenced, and as a result more authoritative and logical. An excellent site.

Allergy and triggers in asthma

http://www.housedustmite.org – a fun site, packed with information that will inform and entertain patients and healthcare professionals. More facts than you ever wished to know about the mites.

http://www.theallergyreport.com – provides guidance on the management of allergic disorders in primary care. This American site provides clear information and is comprehensive and well presented. It is mostly germane to European practice and is evidence based.

http://www.airquality.co.uk – useful for patients whose asthma seems extremely sensitive to changes in air quality, especially those with mixed asthma and chronic obstructive pulmonary disease.

http://www.uksport.gov.uk – provides the latest and most authoritative information on which medications (including non-prescription drugs) are allowed or prohibited by UK national and some international bodies.

Occupational asthma

http://www.nhsplus.nhs.uk – an excellent site, beautifully but simply presented, which contains all the information needed by employers, employees and healthcare professionals regarding occupational asthma.

http://www.agius.com/hew/resource/ocasthma.htm – another good site, designed for healthcare professionals, with good links.

Miscellaneous

http://www.bbc.co.uk/health/asthma – a very good site for patients, and well worth directing newly diagnosed patients to. Information is presented clearly, simply and in depth without being condescending.

http://isaac.auckland.ac.nz – presents the main findings of the ongoing International Study of Asthma and Allergies in Childhood (ISAAC), colourfully and well.

Patient sites

http://www.asthma.org.uk – the National Asthma Campaign's website. Very comprehensive, clear and supportive. Although aimed mainly at patients, many healthcare professionals will find this a valuable site.

http://www.Asthmadirect.com – a useful source of products that some asthma patients may find a help.

http://www.pslgroup.com/asthma.htm – an excellent site for the newly diagnosed patient or carer who wishes to know as much as possible about asthma. Unusually for a patient-oriented site, many recent articles are presented. Although primarily for patients, it has sufficient depth to be useful and interesting to many healthcare professionals as well.

http://www.faqs.org/faqs/medicine/asthma/general-info – and many related sites, all of which can be accessed via this one, providing ongoing dialogue and discussion about all aspects of asthma and its management.

http://www.nhlbisupport.com/asthma/about.html – The Asthma Management Model System is an information management tool designed to facilitate science-based decision-making and evidence-based medicine in long-term asthma management. The system consists of three main components: The Research Mode links to and integrates a variety of searchable databases and other resources. The Education Mode provides immediate access to clinical practice guidelines, an electronic library, continuing education and patient education materials, and teaching/learning tools. The Communication Mode allows you to e-mail the Webmaster and register for updates, and will soon connect to online forums and discussions.

http://www.asthmatool.com – an excellent site, providing clear references to a wide variety of asthma-related topics. It basically provides a mini-search engine from Health on the Net Foundation, a non-profit-making organization that lists sites by their integrity and relevance, so screening out many of the more dubious or commercial sites.

http://www.asthmaexplained.co.uk – a good site for student healthcare professionals or very interested non-medical patients. Quite clear and simple.

http://www.about-asthma.com – good for new patients, but more experienced patients may find this site too simplistic.

http://www.asthma-maintenance.com – good, basic education, clearly presented.

Clinical evidence
Clinical evidence (a compendium of the best available evidence for effective health care, published by the BMJ Publishing Group) can be accessed at http://www.clinicalevidence.org

The Cochrane database can be accessed at http://www.cochrane.org

REFERENCES

PREFACE

1. British Thoracic Society. The British guidelines on asthma management, 1995. Review and position statement. *Thorax* 1997; **52:** S1–S21.

2. National Institutes of Health. *Global Initiatives for Asthma – global strategy for asthma management and prevention.* NHBLI/WHO workshop report. Bethesda, MD: NIH; 1995.

CHAPTER 1

1. International Asthma Management Project. International consensus report on the diagnosis and management of asthma. *Clin Exp Allergy* 1992; **22**(1 supplement): 1–72.

2. Global Initiative for Asthma. *Asthma management and prevention: a practical guide for health care professionals.* Bethesda, MD: GINA, US Department of Health and Human Studies, Public Health Service & National Heart, Lung and Blood Institute, National Institutes of Health, 1998.

3. Sutar A, Hawker C, Seaton A, Peake C. Oilseed rape and bronchial reactivity. *Occup Environ Med* 1990; **52**(9): 575–580.

4. Devereaux G, Ayatohalin T, Ward R et al. Asthma, airways responsiveness and air pollution in two contrasting districts in northern England. *Thorax* 1996; **57:** 109–134.

5. von Mutius E, Martinez F, Fritzch C et al. Prevalence of asthma and atopy in two areas of West and East Germany. *Am J Respir Crit Care Med* 1994; **149:** 61–77.

6. Austin J, Russell G, Adam M et al. Prevalence of asthma and wheeze in the Highlands of Scotland. *Arch Dis Child* 1994; **71:** 211–216.

7. Bradshaw L, Fishwick D, Kemp T et al. Under the volcano: fire, ash and asthma? *N Z Med J* 1997; **110:** 90–91.

8. National Asthma Campaign. Out in the open: a true picture of asthma in the United Kingdom today. *Asthma J* 2001; **6:** 3–14.

9. British Thoracic Society, Scottish Intercollegiate Guidelines Network (SIGN). British Guideline on the management of asthma. *Thorax* 2003; **58** (Suppl I): S1–94.

10. National Institutes of Health. *Global Initiatives for Asthma – global strategy for asthma management and prevention.* NHBLI/WHO workshop report. Bethesda, MD: NIH; 1995.

11. International Study of Asthma and Allergies in Childhood (ISAAC) Steering Committee. Worldwide variation in prevalence of symptoms of asthma, allergic rhinoconjunctivitis, and atopic eczema: ISAAC. *Lancet* 1998; **351:** 1225–1232.

12. Schwartz RS. A new element in the mechanism of asthma. *N Engl J Med* 2002; **346:** 857–858.

CHAPTER 3

1. Ward C, Pavi M, Bish R et al. Airway inflammation, basement membrane thickening and bronchial hyperresponsiveness in asthma. *Thorax* 2002; **57:** 309–316.

2. Panhuysen C, Vonk J, Koeter G et al. Adult patients may outgrow their asthma: a 25 year follow-up study. *Am Rev Respir Crit Care Med* 1997; **155:** 1267–1272.

3. Joint Health Services Unit. *Health Survey for England 1996*. London: Stationery Office; 1998.

4. Joint Health Surveys Unit. *Health Survey for Scotland 1996*. Edinburgh: Stationery Office; 1998.

5. National Asthma Campaign. *National Asthma Audit 1997/98*. London: NAC; 1997.

6. Ernst P, Spitzer W, Suissa S et al. Risk of fatal and near-fatal asthma in relation to inhaled corticosteroid use. *JAMA* 1992; **268:** 3462–3464.

7. Model D. Preventable factors and death certification in death due to asthma. *Respir Med* 1995; **89:** 21–25.

8. Berrill W. Death rate from asthma. *BMJ* 1993; **306:** 854 (letter).

9. National Asthma Campaign. Out in the open: a true picture of asthma in the United Kingdom today. *Asthma J* 2001; **6:** 3–14.

10. Madden V. Survey shows UK's high asthma rates. *Pract Nurse* 1997; **14:** 297.

11. Haahtela T, Jarvinen M, Kara T et al. Comparison of a β_2-agonist, terbutaline, with an inhaled corticosteroid, budesonide, in newly detected asthma. *N Engl J Med* 1991; **325:** 388–392.

12. Juniper E, Kline P, Vanzieleghem M et al. Effect of long-term treatment with an inhaled corticosteroid (budesonide) on airway hyper-responsiveness and clinical asthma in non-steroid-dependent asthmatics. *Am Rev Respir Dis* 1990; **142:** 832–836.

CHAPTER 4

1. Bousquet J. Immunotherapy is clinically indicated in the management of allergic asthma: pro. *Am J Respir Crit Care Med* 2001; **164:** 2139–2140.

2. Franklin Adkinson N. Immunotherapy is clinically indicated in the management of allergic asthma: con. *Am J Respir Crit Care Med* 2001; **164:** 2140–2141.

3. Gotzsche P, Hammerquist C, Burr M. House dust mite control measures in the management of asthma: meta-analysis. *BMJ* 1998; **317:** 1105–1110.

4. Abramson M, Puy R, Weiner J. Is allergen immunotherapy effective in asthma? A meta-analysis of randomised controlled trials. *Am J Resp Crit Care Med* 1995; **151**(4): 969–974.

5. Manocha R, Marks GB, Kenchington P et al. Sahaja yoga in the management of moderate to severe asthma: a randomised controlled trial. *Thorax* 2002; **57:** 110–115.

6. Huntley A, White AR, Ernst E. Relaxation therapies for asthma: a systematic review. *Thorax* 2002; **57:** 127–131.

7. Van Shayck C, Dompeling E, Van Herwaarden C et al. Continuous use of bronchodilator versus use on demand in mild asthma and COPD. *Am J Respir Crit Care Med* 1994; **4**(2): A203.

8. Van Shayck C, Van Herwaarden C, Van Weel C. Asthma control. *Lancet* 1994; **344:** 124 (letter).

9. British Thoracic Society, Scottish Intercollegiate Guidelines Network (SIGN). British Guideline on the management of asthma. *Thorax* 2003; **58** (Suppl I): S1–94.

10. National Institutes of Health. *Global Initiatives for Asthma – global strategy for asthma management and prevention*. NHBLI/WHO workshop report. Bethesda, MD: NIH; 1995.

11. Laitinan L, Laitinan A, Haahtela T. A comparative study of the effects of an inhaled corticosteroid, budesonide, and of a β_2-agonist, terbutaline, on airway inflammation in newly diagnosed asthmatics. *J Allergy Clin Immunol* 1992; **90:** 32–34.

12. Haahtela T, Järvinen M, Kara T et al. Effects of reducing or discontinuing inhaled budesonide in patients with mild asthma. *N Engl J Med* 1994; **331:** 700–705.

13. Dompeling E, Van Schayck C, Moleman J et al. Inhaled beclomethasone improves the cause of asthma and COPD. *Eur Respir J* 1992; **5:** 945–952.

14. Pederson S, Agertoft L. Effect of long-term budesonide treatment on growth, weight and lung function in children with asthma. *Am Rev Respir Dis* 1993; **147:** 265.

15. Ward C, Pavi M, Bish R et al. Airway inflammation, basement membrane thickening and bronchial hyperresponsiveness in asthma. *Thorax* 2002; **57:** 309–316.

16. Juniper E, Kline P, Vanzieleghem M et al. Effect of long-term treatment with an inhaled corticosteroid (budesonide) on airway hyper-responsiveness and clinical asthma in non-steroid-dependent asthmatics. *Am Rev Respir Dis* 1990; **142:** 832–836.

17. Brand P, Kerstjens H, Postma D et al. Long-term multicentre trial in chronic non-specific lung disease: methodology and baseline assessment in adult patients. *Eur Respir J* 1992; **5:** 21–31.

18. Haahtela R, Järvinen M, Kara T et al. Comparison of a β_2-agonist, terbutaline, with an inhaled corticosteroid, budesonide, in newly detected asthma. *N Engl J Med* 1991; **325:** 388–392.

19. Ilais L, Suissa S, Boivin J-F, Ernst P. First treatment with inhaled corticosteroids and the prevention of admissions to hospital for asthma. *Thorax* 1998; **53:** 1025–1029.

20. Agertoft L, Pederson S. Effect of long-term treatment with inhaled budesonide on adult height in children with asthma. *N Engl J Med* 2000; **343:** 1064–1069.

21. Silverstein M, Yunginger J, Reed C et al. Attained adult height after childhood asthma; effect of glucocorticoid therapy. *J Allergy Clin Immunol* 1997; **99**(4): 466–474.

22. Magnussen H, Willenbrock V, Jorres R. Airway responsiveness, lung function and symptoms after cessation of high dose inhaled corticosteroids with bronchial asthma. *Am Rev Respir Dis* 1992; **145:** 498.

23. Juniper E, Kline P, Vanzieleghem M, Hargraves F. Reduction of budesonide after a year of increased use: a randomised controlled trial to evaluate whether improvements in airway responsiveness and clinical asthma are maintained. *J Allergy Clin Immunol* 1991; **87:** 483–489.

24. Redington A, Howarth P. Airway remodelling in asthma. *Thorax* 1997; **52:** 310–312.

25. Greening A, Ind P, Northfield M, Shaw G. Added salmeterol versus higher-dose corticosteroid in asthma patients with symptoms on existing inhaled corticosteroids. *Lancet* 1994; **334:** 219–224.

26. Woolcock A, Lundback B, Ringdal N, Jaques LA. Comparison of the addition of salmeterol to inhaled steroids with doubling of the dose of inhaled steroids. *Am J Respir Crit Care Med* 1996; **153:** 1481–1488.

27. Pauwels R, Lofdahl C-G, Postma D et al for the Formoterol and Corticosteroid Establishing Therapy (FACET) International Study Group. Effect of inhaled formoterol and budesonide on exacerbations of asthma. *N Engl J Med* 1997; **337:** 1405–1411.

28. Shrewsbury S, Pyke S, Britton M. Meta-analysis of increased dose of inhaled steroid or addition of salmeterol in symptomatic asthma (MIASMA). *BMJ* 2000; **103:** 1368–1373.

29. Tasche M, van der Wondon J, Uijen J et al. Randomized placebo-controlled trial of inhaled cromoglycate in 1–4 year old children with moderate asthma. *Lancet* 1997; **350:** 1660–1664.

30. British Thoracic Society. The British guidelines on asthma management, 1995. Review and position statement. *Thorax* 1997; **52:** S1–S21.

31. Hoskins G, Neville R, Smith B, Clark R. Do self-management plans reduce morbidity in patients with asthma? *Br J Gen Pract* 1996; **46:** 169–171.

32. Lahdensuo A, Haahtela T, Herrala J et al. Randomised comparison of guided self management and traditional treatment of asthma over one year. *BMJ* 1996; **312:** 748–752.

33. National Institute of Clinical Excellence. *Inhaler devices for chronic asthma in older children (aged 5–15)*. London: NICE; 2002.

CHAPTER 5

1. Rabe KF, Vermiere PA, Soriano JB, Maier WC. Clinical management of asthma in 1999. The Asthma Insights and Reality in Europe (AIRE) study. *Eur Respir J* 2000; **16:** 802–807.

2. Rickard KA, Stempel DA. Asthma survey demonstrates that the goals of the NHLBI have not been accomplished. *J Allergy Clin Immunol* 1999; **103:** S171.

3. Asher MI, Anderson HR, Stewart AW et al on behalf of the ISAAC Steering Committee. Worldwide variations in the prevalence rates of asthma symptoms: ISAAC. *Eur Respir J* 1998; **12:** 315–335.

4. Burney P, Chinn D, Jarvis D et al. Variations in the prevalence of asthma symptoms, self-reported asthma attacks, and the use of asthma medication in the European Community Respiratory Health Survey (ECRHS). *Eur Respir J* 1996; **9:** 687–695.

5. Action Asthma. *National asthma survey results*. Uxbridge: Allen & Hanbury; 1991.

6. Action Asthma. *Young asthmatics survey*. Uxbridge: Allen & Hanbury; 1993.

7. National Asthma Campaign. *The Impact of Asthma Survey*. London: National Asthma Campaign; 1996.

8. Gruffydd-Jones K, Bell J, Fehrenbach C et al. Understanding patient perceptions of asthma, results of the Asthma Control and Expectations (ACE) Survey. *Int J Clin Pract* 2002; **56:** 89–95.

9. Beasley R, Masoli M. Evidence that therapeutic goals have not been met in asthma. *Prim Care Respir J* 2002; **11**(supplement 1): S3–S6.

10. Lung and Information Agency. *Trends in hospital admissions and deaths from asthma*. Factsheet 2002/1. London: St George's Hospital.

11. Pearson MG, Bucknall CE. *Measuring clinical outcomes in asthma – a patient focused approach*. London: Clinical Effectiveness and Evaluation Unit, Royal College of General Physicians; 1999.

12. British Thoracic Society. BTS guidelines for the management of chronic obstructive pulmonary disease. *Thorax* 1997; **52:** S1–52.

13. Ross D, Sathe B, McDonald J. SWORD '94: surveillance of work-related and occupational respiratory disease in the UK. *Occup Med* 1995; **45:** 175–178.

14. Bosley C, Parry D, Cockrane G. Patient compliance with inhaled medication. Does combing beta-agonists with corticosteroids improve compliance? *Eur Respir J* 1994; **7**(3): 504–509.

15. Avol EL, James Gauderman W, Tan SM et al. Respiratory effects of relocating to areas of differing air pollution levels. *Am J Respir Crit Care Med* 2001; **164:** 2067–2072.

16. British Thoracic Society. Guidelines for the management of asthma in adults. *BMJ* 1990; **301:** 651–653.

17. Podell R. National guidelines for the management of asthma in adults. *Am Fam Phys* 1992; **46**(4): 1189–1196.

18. International Asthma Management Project. International consensus report on the diagnosis and management of asthma. *Clin Exp Allergy* 1992; **22**(1 supplement): 1–72.

19. British Thoracic Society. Guidelines on the management of asthma. *Thorax* 1993; **48**: S1–S24.

20. McGovern V, Crockett A. 1993 BTS guidelines: impact and shortfall 1996. *Asthma J* 1997; **1**(5): 30–31.

21. British Thoracic Society. The British guidelines on asthma management, 1995. Review and position statement. *Thorax* 1997; **52**: S1–S21.

22. British Thoracic Society, Scottish Intercollegiate Guidelines Network (SIGN). British Guideline on the management of asthma. *Thorax* 2003; **58** (Suppl I): S1–94.

23. National Institutes of Health. *Global Initiatives for Asthma – global strategy for asthma management and prevention.* NHBLI/WHO workshop report. Bethesda, MD: NIH; 1995.

24. Bryce F, Neville R, Crombie I et al. Controlled trial of an audit facilitator in diagnosis and treatment of childhood asthma in general practice. *BMJ* 1995; **310**: 838–843.

CHAPTER 6

1. Busse WW. Anti-immunoglubulin E (omalizumab) therapy in allergic asthma. *Am J Respir Crit Care Med* 2001; **164**: S12–S17.

GLOSSARY

A&E – accident and emergency
ACTH – adrenocorticotrophic hormone
AIRE – Asthma Insights and Reality in Europe
BTS – British Thoracic Society
CFC – chlorofluorocarbon
COPD – chronic obstructive pulmonary disease
FACET – Formoterol And Corticosteroid Establishing Therapy (study)
FEV$_1$ – forced expiratory volume in 1 second
FVC – forced vital capacity
GINA – Global Initiative for Asthma
GORD – gastro-oesophageal reflux disease
GP – general practitioner
HFA – hydrofluoroalkane

Ig – immunoglobulin
ISAAC – International Study of Asthma and Allergies in Childhood
LTRA – leukotriene receptor antagonist
MDI – metered-dose inhaler
NHS – National Health Service
NSAID – non-steroidal anti-inflammatory drug
PEF – peak expiratory flow
RAST – radioallergosorbent test
SCIAD – Scottish Confidential Inquiry into Asthma Deaths
SIGN – Scottish Intercollegiate Guidelines Network
Th1/Th2 – T helper cell type 1/type 2
TNF – tumour necrosis factor
VIP – vasoactive inhibitory peptide

LIST OF PATIENT QUESTIONS

Chapter 1

What is asthma?	35
Is asthma very common?	35
Why is asthma becoming more common?	35
Does pollution cause asthma?	35
Can you catch asthma?	35
Can asthma be cured?	36
If I have asthma, will my baby develop it too?	36

Chapter 2

How do I know I've got asthma?	63
How do I know my child has asthma?	63
Why do many people seem to have asthma and hay fever and eczema?	63
Will my child grow out of the asthma?	63

Chapter 4

Why should I need to take inhaled steroids for my asthma – surely it would be better to avoid whatever causes my asthma?	158
I find it very difficult to find the time and money I should be spending in trying to reduce the dust and mite exposure in my house. What should I do to help my daughter who has asthma?	158
How can I tell if my asthma is getting better or worse?	158
Are inhaled steroids safe even in children or if used over a long time?	159
Does it matter if I miss the occasional dose of my regular inhalers?	159
If steroids are so safe, why are sportsmen and women not allowed to use them?	159
How does my doctor or nurse know which treatment is right for me?	159
Will treating my asthma help make the disease go away, or will I need to take treatment all my life?	160
Will I get addicted to any of my treatments?	160

Chapter 6

My son takes a brown puffer twice a day and a blue one when needed, via a spacer. He starts school next week. What should I do about his inhalers?	229
My granny is aged 80 and has asthma. She should take a purple inhaler twice a day and a blue one if she needs it, but she keeps forgetting and tells me they don't work even when she does take them. She is quite breathless most of the time. What should I do?	229
Will there ever be a cure for asthma?	229

INDEX

As asthma is the subject of the book, all index entries refer to asthma unless otherwise indicated. Page numbers in **bold** refer to figures and/or tables.

A

Able Spacer, 236
absenteeism, 70
Accuhaler, 149, **149**
  advantages/disadvantages, 151–152
  disabled patients, 156
  drugs compatible, 235
  use, 150
Action on Smoking and Health (ASH), 241
acupuncture, 92
acute severe asthma, 136–140
  assessment, 137
  children/infants, 137
  complications, 62
  follow-up, 139–140
  life-threatening features, 136, 137
  physical signs, 43
  recognition, 136–137
  symptoms, 42
  treatment, 137–138
    response, 138–139
adolescents, 182–184, 203
adrenal function, steroid effects, 104–105
adults
  diagnosis in, 59–61, 185
    differential, **54**
  disease loss, 76
  exercise-induced asthma, 203
  management, 185–186
    plan, 186
  natural history, 68
  nebulizers, 154–155
  referral, 186
  risk factors, 58
    childhood asthma, 60–61, 66, 67–68
    disease persistence, 76
  stepwise approach, 124–125
  symptoms, 41
  treatment, 185
    steroid doses, 100
  triggers, 185
A&E departments, 213, 216
  see also hospital admissions
AeroChamber, 144

Aerohaler, 149
  advantages/disadvantages, 152–153
  drugs compatible, 235
  use, 151
Aerolizer, 149
  advantages/disadvantages, 153
  drugs compatible, 235
  use, 151
aetiological factors, 6–16
age
  allergens exposure, 33
  deterioration, 76–77
  presentation, 29
  prevalence, **18, 22**
  sensitization, 27, 33
  steroid use, 99–100
airway disease, 201
allergens, 6–16
  avoidance, 88–89
    improving, 225
  definition, 6
  exposure age, 33
  house mite, 7–8
  information resources, 244
  pathology, 30
  sensitization see sensitization
  see also triggers
allergic asthma, 5
  molecular biology advances, clinical
    benefit, 226
  pathology, 30–31
  treatment, 119–120
  see also allergens; atopic asthma
allergic granulomatosis, 114
allergic reaction, 6
allergy
  detection, 51–52, 87–88
  in diagnosis, 44
  Internet testing, 52–53
  therapy, 87–92
alternative therapy, 92–93
American College of Allergy, Asthma and
    Immunology, 243
American Lung Association, 243
aminophylline
  acute severe asthma, 138
  brand names, 233
  side-effects, 138
animals, 89
  aetiological role, 8–9
  allergens, **9,** 89

animals (*Cont'd*)
  avoidance, 89
antibiotics, 119
anticholinergic agents, 117–118
  brand names, 232
  children, 118
  elderly patients, 118
  future, 224
  ipratropium *see* ipratropium bromide
  mechanism, 117
  obstructive airway disease (mixed), 191
  side-effects, 117
  use, 118
antihistamines, 119–120
antioxidants
  aetiological role, 16
  increasing prevalence, 26
anxiety, 212
  aetiological role, 14
  management of patients, 201
armed forces, 195
aspirin, 207
  aetiological role, 14–15
associated conditions, 55
asthma
  acute severe *see* acute severe asthma
  allergic *see* allergic asthma
  atopic *see* atopic asthma
  brittle *see* brittle asthma
  definition, 4–5
  effects of, 69–73, **70**
  exercise-induced *see* exercise-induced
      asthma
  future prospects, 223–230
  intrinsic, 5–6
  mild, 99
  natural history, 66–77
  non-allergic asthma, 13–14, 34
  occupational *see* occupational asthma
  patient questions *see* patient questions
  refractive, 211–213
  severe chronic, **131**
  travel and, 208–209
Asthma and Allergy Foundation of America,
    242
Asthma Control and Expectations Survey,
    168
atopic asthma, 5
  manifestations, 55
  treatment, 114
  see also allergic asthma
audit
  areas, 218–219
  changes, 220–221
  cycle, **219**
  data analysis, 218, 220
  data collection, 219–220
  patient management, 217–222
  principles, 217–218

sophisticated, 221–222
Autohaler, 147, **148**
  disabled patients, 156–157
  drugs compatible, 235

B

β_2-agonists, 95–98
  adults, 185
  advantages, 110
  alternative drugs, 98, 118
  brand names, 231, 232
  children, 181
  cough variant asthma, 206
  disadvantages, 110–111
  excessive use, 97
  exercise-induced asthma, 203–204
  inhaled, 96, 97, 151, 152
    acute severe asthma, 137
    inhalers compatible, 231–234
  long-acting, 110–112
  lung function decline, 97
  mechanism of action, 95
  morbidity/mortality, 97
  obstructive airway disease (mixed), 191
  oral, 96, 97, 112
  peak flow rate response, **48,** 97
  pregnancy and, 187
  short-acting, 95–97
  side-effects, 96, 112
  steroid use with, 98, 109–110, 111, 112
  teenagers, 183–184
  toddlers, 179
  toxicity, 110–111
  types, 97, 110, 112
  use, 95–96, 109
    frequency, 96
    in practice, 111
  see also specific drugs
Babyhaler, 144
beclometasone, 111
  brand names, 231–232, 237
  salmeterol use with, 109
behavioural effects of steroids, 106
birch pollen allergy syndrome, 16
blood tests, diagnosis, 51–52
bone metabolism, steroid effects, 105
breath-actuated devices (BADs), 140,
    147–148
  advantages/disadvantages, 148
  disabled patients, 156
  drugs compatible, 231–234, 235
  types, 147
  use, 147–148
breathing exercises, 92–93
British Lung Foundation, 240
British Thoracic Society (BTS)
  guidelines, 17, 214, 215

British Thoracic Society (BTS) (*Cont'd*)
    drug administration, 98
    management regimens, 123
    stepwise approach, 124–127, **126**
    see also Scottish Intercollegiate Guidelines
        Network (SIGN)
brittle asthma
    diagnosis, 188
    management, 188–190
        drug treatment, 188–189
    referral, 190
    triggers, 188
    type I, 188–189
    type II, 188, 189
bronchodilators
    β_2-agonists *see* β_2-agonists
    brittle asthma, 189
    children, 181
    elderly patients, 196
    future, 224
    infants, 176
    nebulizers, 154–155
    obstructive airway disease (mixed), 191
    teenagers, 183
    theophyllines *see* theophyllines
    toddlers, 179
    see also specific drugs
bronchospasm, causes, 6, 8
BTS *see* British Thoracic Society (BTS)
budesonide
    brand names, 232, 233, 237
    nebulizers, 154

C

carer burden, 70–71
cat allergy, **9,** 89
cataract, steroid effects, 105
chest infections, 206–207
chest X-ray in diagnosis, 50–51
chickenpox, 122
children, 55–59
    acute severe asthma, 137
    cromogens, 117
    development of adult disease, 56–59, 64
        prediction, 67, 76
        risk factors, 58, 66, 67–68
        risk reduction, 58–59
    diagnosis, 47, 180
        differential, **54**
    exercise-induced asthma, 202–203
    management, 86, 180–182
        anticholinergic drugs, 118
        formoterol fumarate (eformoterol), 111
        medication, 181
        nebulizers, 155
        plan, 182
        salmeterol xinafoate, 111

        spacers, 146–147
        steroids, 100, 106, 159
        see also individual treatments
    natural history, 66–69
        intervention effects, 66–67
    patient questions, 64, 229
    patient referral, 182
    patient review, 216
    school and, 181–182, 229
    stepwise approach, 124–125
    symptoms, 41
    teacher role, 182
    teenagers, 182–184
    toddlers, 178–180
    triggers, 180–181
    see also infants
chiropractic therapy, 92
chloride channel blockers, 225
chlorofluorocarbons (CFCs), 142–143
chronic obstructive pulmonary disease
    (COPD), 190
    differences, **60,** 61–62
    differential diagnosis, 191
        importance, 62
    management, 119, 190–193
    misdiagnosis, 61
    smoking risk, 76
    symptoms, 191
    treatment, 118
        future, 224
Churg–Strauss syndrome, 114
Ciclesonide, 224
ciclosporin, 224
classification, 16–27
Clickhaler, 149
    advantages/disadvantages, 152
    disabled patients, 156
    drugs compatible, 235
    use, 150
clinical features, 40–44
cockroaches, aetiological role, 9
community practitioners, 173
compliance, 198–200
    accidental non-compliance, 199
    deliberate non-compliance,
        198–199
    elderly patients, 229
    factors affecting, 198
    improvement, 198, 199–200
complications, 62
control
    criteria, 86–97
    physical signs, 43
    poor
        complications, 62
        physical signs, 43
        prognosis, 69
        signs, 222
prognosis, 69

costs, 65–78, 73–77
    direct medical resources, 74
    indirect, 74
    NHS, 73
    non-medical resources, 74
    social, 70
cough
    association, 56
    causes, 67
    steroid side-effects, 104
    variant, 205–208
        differential diagnosis, 206
cromogens, 116–117
    children, 117
    inhaled, 98–99
    mechanism, 116–117
    types, 116
    use, 117
cromoglicate, 116
    brand names, 232, 233, 237
    nebulizers, 154
    use, 117
cure, 36, 229
cycling, 11

D

depression, 201
desensitization (immunotherapy), 88
deterioration
    age, 76–77
    improvement, 76
    patient questions, 158
    patient recognition, 133
diagnosis, 37–64, **49**
    adults, 185
    brittle asthma, 188
    children, 47, 180
    differential, 44, 53–55
    elderly patients, 60, 195
    exercise-induced asthma, 202–203
    guidelines, 216
    incorrect, 59, 62, 211
    infants, 47, 176
    investigations, 45–53, 60
    obstructive airway disease (mixed),
        190–191
    occupational asthma, 194
    patient questions, 64–65
    primary care, 174–175
    teenagers, 182–183
    toddlers, 178
diet, 92
    aetiological role, 15–16, 16, 27
    hypersensitivity reaction, 16
    prevalence and, 23–24, 26
disabled patients, 156
Diskhaler (Diskus), 149
    advantages, 153
    disadvantages, 153
    drugs compatible, 235
    use, 151
disodium cromoglicate see cromoglicate
district nurse, 173
domestic hygiene, 8, 23, 25
drug therapy, 94–122, 231–237
    addiction, 160
    antibiotics, 119
    anticholinergics see anticholinergic agents
    antihistamines, 119–120
    bronchodilators see bronchodilators
    competitive sports, 204, **205**
    compliance see compliance
    cromogens see cromogens
    delivery devices see inhaler devices;
        nebulizers
    future, 224–225
    inhaled see inhaled drugs
    leukotriene antagonists see leukotriene
        receptor antagonists (LTRAs)
    manufacturers' designs, 235–236
    pregnancy and, 187
    primary care, 121, 175
    steroids see steroids
    theophyllines see theophyllines
    types, 95
    see also specific drugs
dry powdered devices, 140, 149–153
    advantages/disadvantages, 151–153
    disabled patients, 156
    drugs compatible, 235–236
    loading required, 149, 150–151
    preloaded, 149, 150
    use, 150–151

E

ear problems, 94
Easi-Breathe, 147, **148**
    advantages, 148
    disabled patients, 156
    drugs compatible, 235
eczema, 64
eformoterol see formoterol fumerate
    (eformoterol)
elderly patients
    anticholinergic agents, 118
    compliance, 229
    diagnosis, 59, 195
    management, 156, 195–196
    nebulizers, 156
    referral, 196
    review of patients, 216
    symptoms, 41
    triggers, 196
    vaccinations, 93–94

emotional burden, 70
environmental effects
  development, 27
  indoor environment, 23, 24–25
  outdoor environment, 25–26
  pollution *see* pollution
  risk reduction, 210
  see also allergens
euphemisms, 56
European Respiratory Society (ERS), 242
exacerbations, 86
examination, 60
exercise
  advice, 91
  aetiological role, 10–11
    see also exercise-induced asthma
  tests in diagnosis, 47
exercise-induced asthma
  adolescent, 203
  adults, 203
  children, 202–203
  diagnosis, 202–203
  management, 202
    long-term, 204
  sportsmen/women, 203, 204
  steroid use, 99
  treatment, 111, 203–204
extrinsic, 5
eyes, steroid effects, 105

F

factors, 4
family burden, 70–71
family history, 44
family size, 8
fluticasone
  brand names, 232
  nebulizers, 154
flying, 208–209
forced expiratory volume in 1 second
    (FEV$_1$), 47, 49–50
Formoterol And Corticosteroid Establishing
    Therapy (FACET) study, 109–110
formoterol fumarate (eformoterol), 110
  brand names, 232, 233
  children, 111
fungi, 9
furosemide (frusemide), 225

G

gastro-oesophageal reflux disease (GORD),
    94
  management, 201
The General Practice Airways Group
    (GPIAG), 239–240
genetics, 27, 28–29, 226–227

gene testing, 52
  patient questions, 36
GINA classification, 4, 17
  management and, 123

H

hay fever, 63
health visitors, 173
histamine, 16
hoarseness of voice, 104
hospital admissions, **169**, 169–170
  A&E departments, 213, 216
  see also specialist referral
house dust mites, **7**
  aetiological role, 7–8
  allergens, 8, 226
  exposure reduction, 90
  optimal conditions, 90
  patient questions, 158
hydrofluoroalkane (HFA), 142–143
hygiene (domestic)
  aetiological role, 8
  prevalence effects, 23, 25
hypersensitivity reaction, 16
hypnosis, 92

I

immune hypothesis, 24, 26
immune system, steroid effects, 106
immunization *see* vaccinations
immunoglobulin (Ig) E levels
  in diagnosis, 51, 52–53
  future treatments, 225
immunology, 226
  see also allergy
immunomodulatory treatment, 224–225
immunotherapy (desensitization), 88
incidence, 19–23, **20, 21**
indomethacin, 224
infants, 178–180
  acute severe asthma, 137
  diagnosis, 47, 176
    differential, 53–54, **54**
  factors contributing to asthma in, 210
  management, 176–178
  medication, 176–177
    bronchodilators, 176
    steroids, 177
  parental considerations, 177–178
  recurrent wheezing, causes, **54**
  referral, 178
  stepwise approach, 125–127
  symptoms, 41
  triggers, 176
  see also children

inflammation
 airway, 33–34
 cascade, 32–33
 pathology, 30–31
 persistence, 34
 role, 32–33
 symptoms, 41–42
influenza vaccination, 93
information resources, 239–246
 allergens, 244
 occupational, 245
 patient sites, 245–246
 triggers, 244
inhaled drugs
 β₂-agonists *see* β₂-agonists
 delivery devices *see* inhaler devices;
  nebulizers
 dose missing, 159
 steroids *see* steroids
inhaler devices, 140–157, 231–237
 breath-actuated *see* breath-actuated devices
  (BADs)
 choice, 140–141
 dry powdered *see* dry powdered devices
 infants, 177
 manufacturers' designs, 235–236
 metered-dose *see* metered-dose inhaler
  (MDI)
 spacers *see* spacers
 see also specific devices
International Consensus Report on diagnosis
  and management, 4
The International Primary Respiratory Care
  Group (IPCRG), 242
International Study of Asthma and Allergies
  in Childhood (ISAAC), 17
intrinsic asthma, 5–6
ipratropium bromide, 117
 acute severe asthma, 138
 brand names, 232, 233, 237
 exercise-induced asthma, 204
 nebulizers, 154

L

leukotriene receptor antagonists (LTRAs),
  112–114
 adults, 185
 advantages, 113–114
 brand names, 233
 children, 181
 cough variant asthma, 206
 disadvantages, 113–114
 exercise-induced asthma, 204
 inhaled, 99
 mechanism, 112–113
 pregnancy, 187
 side-effects, 113, 114

teenagers, 183
toddlers, 179
use, 109, 113
The Lung and Asthma Information Agency,
  241
lung damage, 77
lung function decline, 66, 76, 97
 forced expiratory volume in 1 second
  (FEV₁), 47, 49–50
 peak flow *see* peak flow rate

M

magnesium sulfate, 224
management, 79–160, 161–222
 adult, 185–186
 aims, 69, 86–87
 assessment, 167–169
  individual patients, 170–171
  international comparisons, **168,**
   168–169
  quality-of-life questionnaires, 171
  UK, 167–168
  see also audit
 associated factors, 94
 brittle asthma, 188–190
 children, 86, 178–182
 compliance *see* compliance
 criteria of care, 171
 difficult asthma, 197
 elderly patients, 156, 195–196
 exercise-induced asthma, 202–205
 guidelines/protocols, 214–217
  improvement, 220–221
 infants, 176–178
 mixed obstructive airway disease, 190–193
 newly diagnosed patient, 172
  follow-up, 172–173
 occupational asthma, 193–195
 outcome measures, 170–171
 patients with other diseases, 201
 pregnancy and, 186–188
 primary care clinicians, 173–174
 problems, 176
 refractive asthma, 211–213
 regimens, 123
 self *see* self-management plans
 smoking, 200–201
 stepwise approach *see* stepwise approach
 teenagers, 182–184
 troublesome symptoms, 197, 205–208
 types of asthma, 174–176
 see also treatment
mechanism, 30–34, **31, 32**
medical history in diagnosis, 44, 59
menstrual cycle, 207–208
metered-dose inhaler (MDI), 140, 141–143
 advantages, 141–142

metered-dose inhaler (MDI) (*Cont'd*)
  children, 181
  disabled patients, 156
  disadvantages, 142
  drugs compatible, 231–234, 237
  examples, **141**
  propellants, 142–143
  use, 142
methotrexate, 122, 224
microclimate, 26
mild asthma, 99
molecular biology, 226
mometasone, 100, 107, 224
  brand names, 232
montelukast, 113
  brand names, 233
mood, 14
morbidity measures, 222
mortality, **71**, 71–72, **169**, 169–170
  β$_2$-agonists, 97
  decline, 170
  factors to avoid, **73**
  patient risk, 72–73
  steroids, 72
mould, 9
mycohenolat, 225

N

The National Asthma Campaign, 239
  Impact of Asthma Survey, 168
  UK prevalence, 17–18
National Asthma Survey, 167
National Health Service (NHS) costs, 73
National Institutes of Health (NIH), 242
  Global Initiative for Asthma (GINA), 4,
    17, 123
National Respiratory Training Centre, 240
natural history, 65–78
  adults, 68
  children, 66–69
NebuChamber, 144
  drugs compatible, 232, 236
Nebuhaler, 144
  drugs compatible, 236
nebulizers, 140, 153–155
  acute severe asthma, 139
  adults, 155–156
  advantages/disadvantages, 154
  children, 155
  choice, 155–157
  disabled patients, 156
  economics, 155
  elderly patients, 156
  home use, 154–155
  mechanism, 153
  obstructive airway disease (mixed), 192
  side-effects, 154

  use, 154
  weaning, 155
nedocromil sodium, 116
  brand names, 232
  exercise-induced asthma, 204
  use, 117
nitrogen oxides, 12
nocturnal symptoms, 15, 222
  β$_2$-agonists, 111
  cough variant asthma, 206
  theophyllines, 114
non-allergic asthma
  mechanism, 34
  triggers, 13–14
non-pharmacological treatment, 92–94
nose problems, 94
Novolizer, 149, 151, 153
  drugs compatible, 232, 236

O

obstructive airway disease (mixed)
  diagnosis, 190–191
  management, 190–193
    drug treatment, 191–192
    referral, 192–193
    triggers, 191
occupational asthma, 13
  causes, **14**, 193
  diagnosis, 194
  information resources, 245
  management, 193–194
  prevalence, 193
  prognosis, 76
  triggers, 13
    avoidance, 91
oilseed rape, 10, **10**
omalizumab, 225
Optimiser, 144
oral candidiasis, 104
orciprenaline, 97
  brand names, 231
osteoporosis, 120
otitis media, 55, 94
overdiagnosis, 59
oxitropium, 117
  brand names, 232, 237
oxygen
  acute severe asthma, 137, 139
  management, 119
ozone, 12

P

paediatric liaison nurse, 174
parent burden, 70–71
  infants, 177–178
  toddlers, 180

particulates
  aetiological role, 11
  increasing prevalence, 25
passive smoking, 14
pathology, 30–31
patient denial, management, 197
patient questions
  causes/aetiological, 35–36
  children, 63, 229
  deterioration, 158
  diagnosis, 63
  genetics, 36
  house dust mites, 158
  pollution, 35
  prevalence, 35
  treatment, 158–160
    steroids, 158, 159
patient review, 216–217
patient symptom variation, 40
peak flow rate, 45–47, **49**
  β$_2$-agonist response, **48,** 97
  meters, **45,** 50
  non-asthmatic subjects, 47
  patient monitoring, 133, 134
    role, 135–136
  readings, **46**
  steroid response, **48**
Personal Action Plan, **130**
pets *see* animals
pharmacists, 174
phosphodiesterases, 225
physiotherapy
  management clinicians, 174
  role, 94
pneumococcal vaccination, 93–94
pollen, **9**
  aetiological role, 9
  increasing prevalence, 25
pollution
  advice, 91–92
  aetiological role, 11–12, **12**
  increasing prevalence, 23, 24–25
  patient questions, 35
  role in severity, 12–13
practice nurse, 173
prediction in newborn, 29–30
pregnancy
  drugs, 187
  infant asthma and, 210
  management, 186–188
    plan, 187
  referral, 187–188
  review of patients, 216
  triggers, 186–187
premature birth, 30
presentation age, 29
prevalence, 16–27
  age-specific, **18, 22**
  decreased, 8

increasing, **22,** 23
  patient questions, 35
  reasons, 23–24
  theories, 23–27, **24**
international comparisons, **18**
locations, 19
patient questions, 35
race, 29
rural areas, 11–12, 26–27
sex, 29
UK, 17–19, 19
urban areas, 11–12, 26–27
prevention, primary, 209–210
primary care
  diagnosis, 174–175
  drug therapy, 175
    oral steroids, 121
prognosis, 66–77
  control, 69
  occupational role, 76
  smoking effects on, 76
prostaglandin E, 225
psychosocial factors, 74–75
  management of patients, 201
pulmonary function, 106
Pulvinal, 149
  advantages/disadvantages, 152
  drugs compatible, 236
  use, 150
purpura, 105

Q

quality-of-life questionnaires, 171
QUIT, 241

R

race effects, 29
radioallergosorbent (RAST) test, 51–52
refractive asthma, 211–213
remission, 108
Respiratory Education and Training Centres 240
respiratory failure, chronic, 119
respiratory infections
  aetiological role, 206–207
  risks, 76
revatropate, 224
review of patients, 216–217
rhinitis, 114
running, 11
rural areas, 11–12, 26–27

S

salbutamol (albuterol), 97
  acute severe asthma, 138, 139

salbutamol (albuterol) (*Cont'd*)
  brand names, 231, 233, 237
  nebulizer, 139
salmeterol xinafoate, 110
  beclometasone use with, 109
  brand names, 232, 237
  children, 111
  steroid use with, 110
school, 181–182
  patient questions, 229
school nurse, 174
Scottish Intercollegiate Guidelines Network
      (SIGN)
  guidelines, 17, 214, **215**
    drug administration, 98
    management regimens, 123
    stepwise approach, 124–129, **126**
see also British Thoracic Society
self-management plans, 130–136
  adults, 186
  benefits, 132–133
  brittle asthma, 189
  children, 182
  deterioration recognition, 133
  elderly patients, 196
  examples, **130, 131,** 136
  infants, 177
  obstructive airway disease (mixed), 192
  occupational asthma, 194–195
  patient response to worsening, 133, 134
  peak flow monitoring, 133, 134
    role, 135–136
  pregnancy, 187
  primary care, 175
  severe chronic, **131**
  steroid access, 134
    type, 135
    use, 135
  teenagers, 184
  toddlers, 180
sensitization, 8
  age, 27, 33
severe chronic asthma, **131**
sex bias, 29
SIGN *see* Scottish Intercollegiate Guidelines
      Network (SIGN)
sinusitis treatment, 119
skin, steroid effects, 105
skin prick tests
  diagnosis, 51
  usefulness, 87–88
sleep disturbance, 69–70
smoking, 91, 200–201
  passive, 14
  presentation/management, 62–63
  prognosis, 76
  quitting, 201
  risk of diseases, 76
socioeconomic factors, 27

sodium cromoglicate, 204
Spacehaler, 144
  drugs compatible, 236
spacers, 143–147
  advantages/disadvantages, 144–145
  care of, 146
  children, 146–147
  choice, 145
  disabled patients, 156
  drugs compatible, 231–234, 235–236
  large-volume, 143–144, 145, 236
  medium-volume, 144, 145, 235–236
  obstructive airway disease (mixed), 192
  small-volume, 144, 145–146, 236
  use, 146
specialist referral, 52
  adults, 186
  children, 182
  elderly patients, 196
  guidelines, 216
  infants, 178
  obstructive airway disease (mixed),
      192–193
  pregnancy, 187–188
  teenagers, 184
  toddlers, 180
see also hospital admissions
Spinhaler, 144, 149
  advantages, 153
  disadvantages, 153
  drugs compatible, 236
  use, 151
spirometry in diagnosis, 47, 50
sportsmen/women, 203, 205
stepwise approach, 174–175
  BTS/SIGN, 124–127, **126**
  changing steps, 127
    risks, 129
  initial therapy, 124
  no response to, 128
  stepping down, 127–128, 128–129
    reasons, 129
  stepping up, 128
  use, 127–129
steroids
  acute severe asthma, 137
  additional treatments, 109–110
  adults, 185
  age considerations, 99–100
  airway remodelling effects, 108
  β_2-agonist use with, 98, 109–110, 111, 112
  benefits, 102
  brand names, 231–232
  brittle asthma, 188–189, 189
  children, 105, 106–107, 181
    benefits, 108
    growth effects, 106
    oral use, 121
  compliance, 199–200

steroids (*Cont'd*)
  contraindications, 99
  dose, 100, 106–107
    increased, 109–110
    maintenance, 101
    response, 103
    tapering, 121
  effectiveness, 101–102
  future, 224
  home use, 134, 135
  infants, 177
  inhaled, 98–99, 99–108, 151, 152
    nebulizers, 154
    types, 107
  initial use, 102–103
  lung function decline, 66, 76, 77
  mechanism, 101
  mortality, 72
  obstructive airway disease (mixed), 191
  oral, 120–122
    disease risk, 122
    precautions, 120
    vaccinations, 122
  patient questions, 158, 159
  peak flow rate response, **48**
  pulmonary function, 106
  remission, 108
  safety, 107, 159
  side-effects, 103–104, 120
    adrenal function, 104–105
    behavioural changes, 106
    bone metabolism, 105, 120
    eye problems, 105
    metabolic, 120
    skin problems, 105, 120
    systemic, 104–105
  teenagers, 184
  toddlers, 179
sulfur dioxide
  aetiological role, 11, 12
  increasing prevalence, 25
swimming, 11
Swindon Asthma Group
  mission statement, 87, 170
  self-management plan, **131**
symptoms
  acute severe asthma, 42
  adults, 41
  causes, 41–42
  children, 41
  elderly patients, 41
  infants, 41
  patient variation, 40
  short-term increase, 127
  significance, 42
  troublesome, 197
  type determination from, 43
  usual, 40
synonyms, 56

T

teenagers, 182–184, 203
terbutaline, 97
  brand names, 231, 237
  brittle asthma, 189
theophyllines, 114–116
  adults, 185
  blood level, 115–116
  brand names, 233
  children, 181
  cough variant asthma, 206
  disadvantages, 114
  dose, 114
  elderly patients, 196
  half-life, 116
  interactions, 116
  intravenous administration, 115
  mechanism, 114
  obstructive airway disease (mixed), 191
  pregnancy, 187
  side-effects, 115
  teenagers, 184
  toddlers, 179
  use, 109, 114–115
third-line therapy, 118
throat irritation, 104
tiotropium, 224
toddlers, 178–180
  see also children; infants
traffic, aetiological role, **12**
transmission, 35–36
travel, 208–209
treatment, 79–160
  acute severe asthma, 136–140
  additional, 109–110
  adults, 100, 124–125, 155–156, 185
  allergen avoidance/reduction, 88–89, 90–91
  allergy therapy, 87–92
    desensitization, 88
  brittle asthma, 188–189
  children, 100, 108, 118, 124–125, 155, 181
  choice, 122–129
  compliance *see* compliance
  cost, 157
  diet, 92
  disabled patients, 156
  drugs *see* drug therapy
  elderly patients, 156, 196
  exacerbations, 86
  exercise and, 91, 203–204
  future, 223–230
    specific therapies, 227
  incorrect, 211
  infants/toddlers, 125–127, 176–177, 179
  inhalers *see* inhaler devices
  mild asthma, 123
  moderate asthma, 123

treatment (*Cont'd*)
  nebulizers *see* nebulizers
  non-pharmacological, 92–94
  obstructive airway disease (mixed),
      191–192
  oxygen, 119, 137
  patient questions, 158–160
  pharmacological *see* drug therapy
  preventive, 86, 98–99
  response to
      diagnostic role, 44
      lack of, 128, 211–213
  selection, 122–129
  self-management plans *see* self-
      management plans
  severe asthma, 123
  step approach *see* stepwise approach
  symptom increase, short-term, 127
  teenagers, 183–184
  third-line therapies, 118
  trigger avoidance, 87–92, 211, 225
  see also management; *specific treatments*
triamcinolone, 224
triggers, 6–16
  adults, 185
  avoidance, 87–92, 211
      improving, 225
  brittle asthma, 188
  children, 180–181
  common, 6
  definition, 6
  elderly patients, 196
  infants, 176
  information resources, 244
  non-allergenic, 13–14
  obstructive airway disease (mixed), 191
  occupational, 13
  pregnancy, 186–187
  primary care, 175
  teenagers, 183
  toddlers, 178–179
  see also allergens
Turbohaler, 149, **149**
  advantages, 152
  disabled patients, 156
  disadvantages, 152
  drugs compatible, 236

use, 150
Twisthaler, 150
  drugs compatible, 232, 236
types, 5–6, 140
  differentiation in treatment, 237
  symptom differences, 43
  see also individual types

U
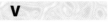

UK prevalence, 17–19, 19
underdiagnosis, 58
urban areas, 11–12, 26–27

V

vaccinations, 26, 93–94
  patients on oral steroids, 122
vasoactive inhibitory peptide (VIP), 224
viral infection, 92
  association, **57**
  as trigger, 6–7
Volumatic, 144, **147**
  drugs compatible, 236

W

weather, 25
wheezing
  association, 56, **57**
  causes, 67
wheezy bronchitis, 56
World Health Organization (WHO), 242

Y

yoga, 92–93
Young Asthmatics Survey, 167–168

Z

zafirlukast, 113
  brand names, 233
  side-effects, 113